THE AUSTRALIAN Women's Weekly

MEDITERRANEAN

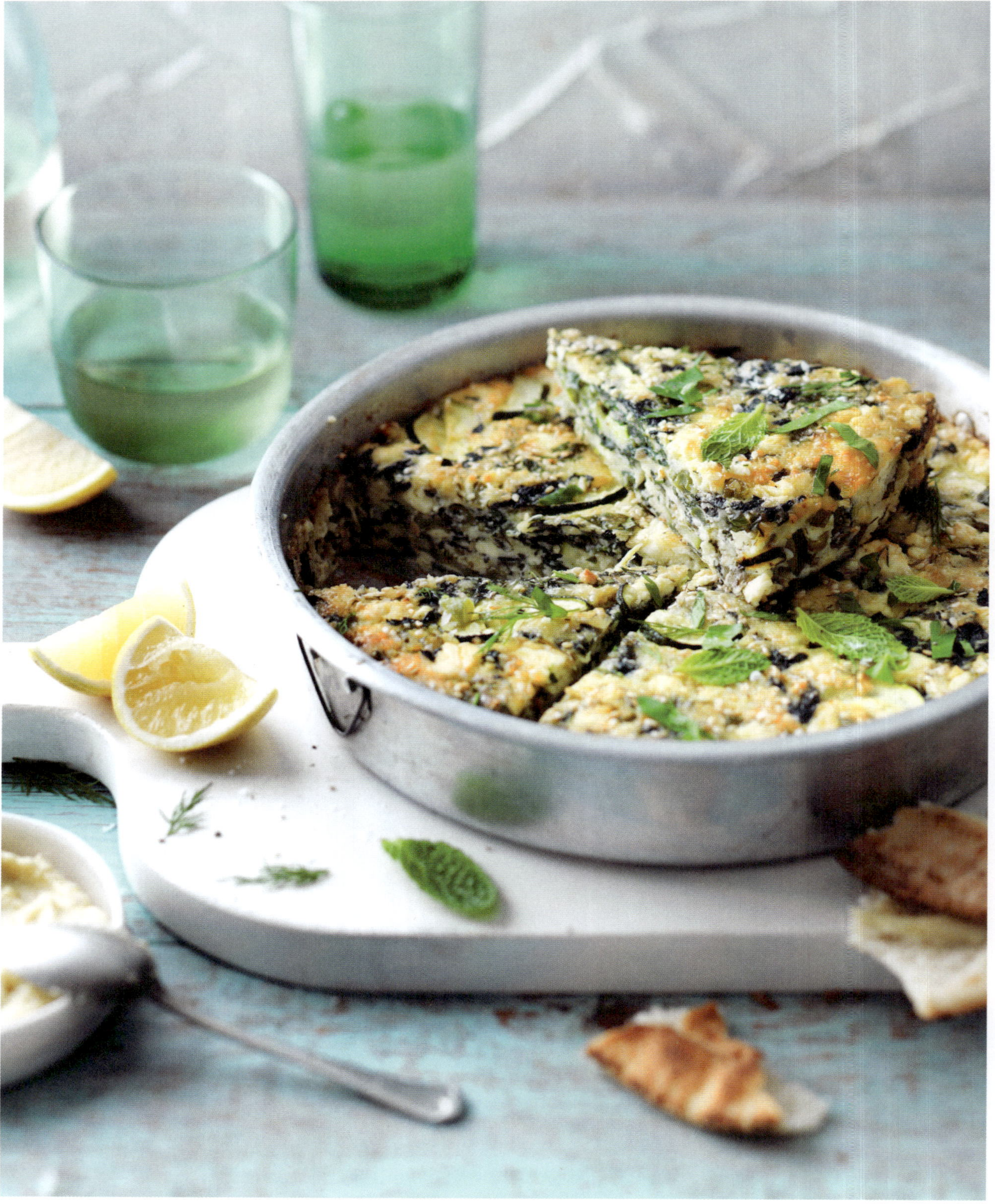

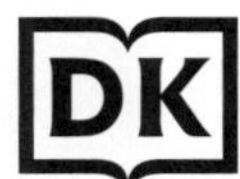

THE AUSTRALIAN Women's Weekly

MEDITERRANEAN

FRESH, HEALTHY
EVERYDAY RECIPES

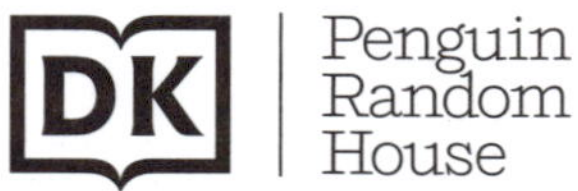

Project Editor Emma Hill
Project Designer Alison Shackleton
Editorial Assistant Kiron Gill
US Editor Nathalie Mornu
US Consultant Renee Wilmeth
Jacket Designer Alison Donovan
Jackets Coordinator Lucy Philpott
Production Editor David Almond
Senior Producer Luca Bazzoli
Creative Technical Support Sonia Charbonnier
Managing Editor Dawn Henderson
Managing Art Editor Alison Donovan
Art Director Maxine Pedliham
Publishing Director Katie Cowan

Photographer Louise Lister
Stylist Emma Knowles
Photochefs Peta Dent, Amal Webster

First American Edition, 2020
Published in the United States by DK Publishing
1450 Broadway, Suite 801, New York, NY 10018

21 22 23 24 25 10 9 8 7 6 5 4 3 2 1
001–324523–May/2021

Published in Great Britain by Dorling Kindersley Limited

A catalog record for this book is available from the Library of Congress.
ISBN 978-0-7440-4071-5

Printed and bound in China

For the curious
www.dk.com

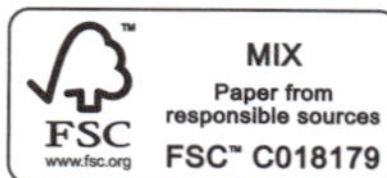

This book was made with Forest Stewardship Council ™ certified paper— one small step in DK's commitment to a sustainable future. For more information go to **www.dk.com/our-green-pledge**

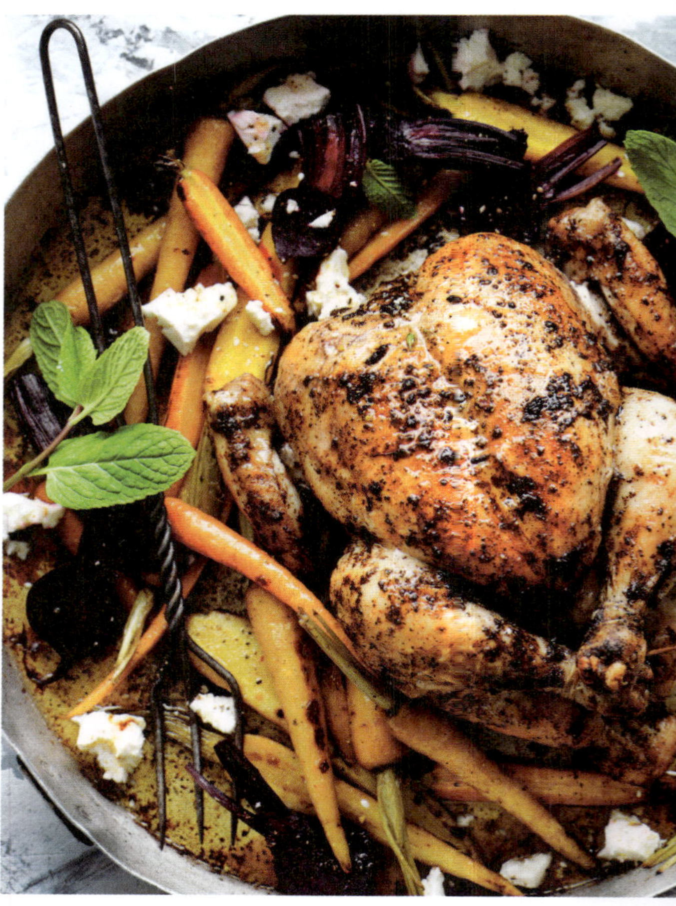

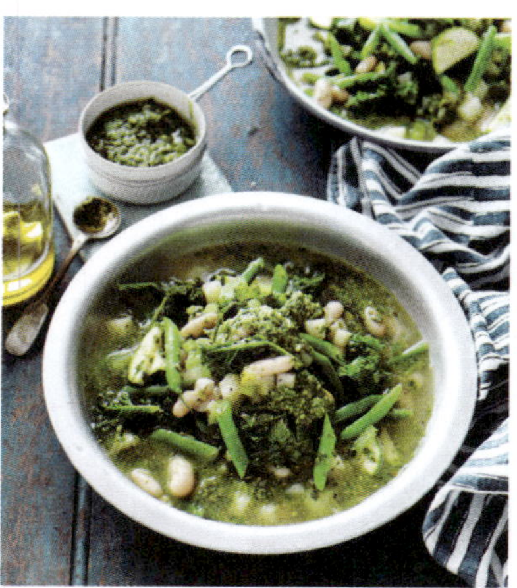

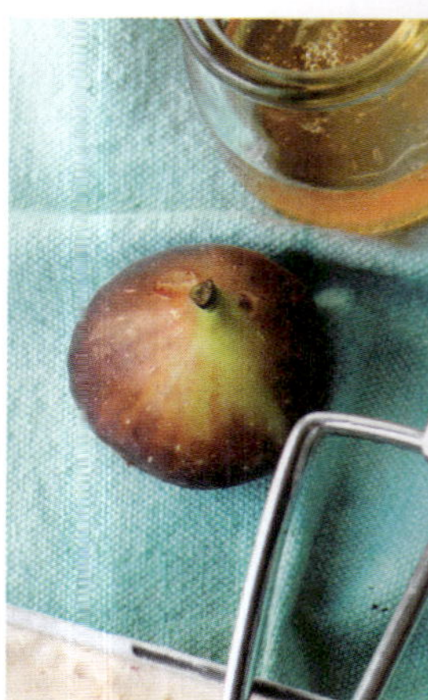

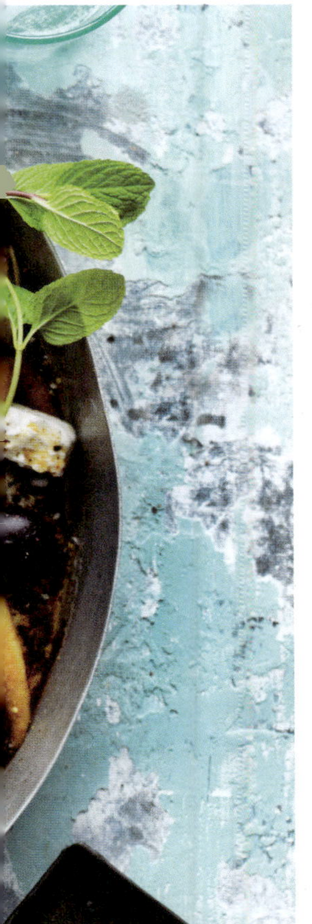
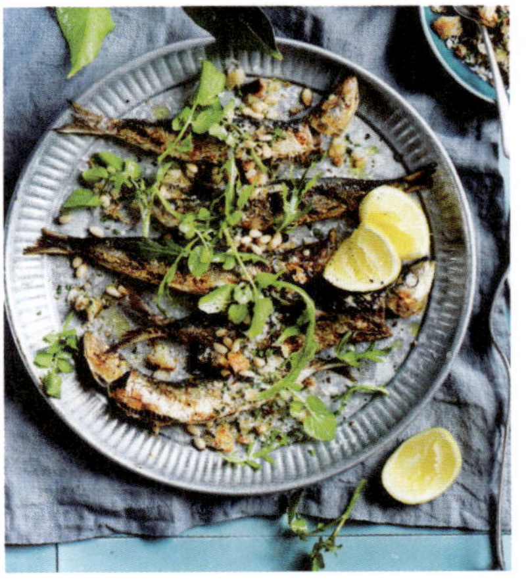
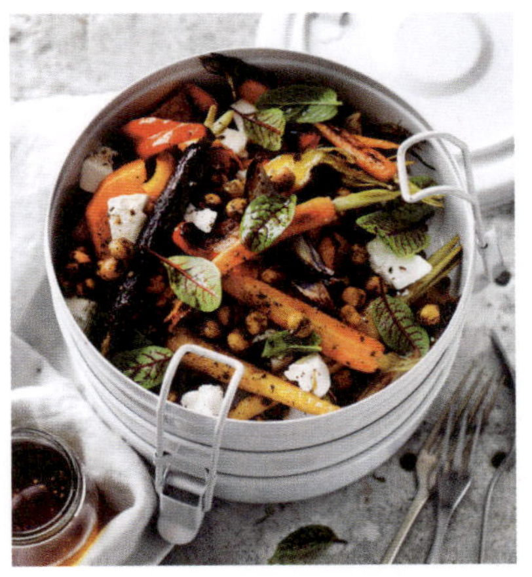
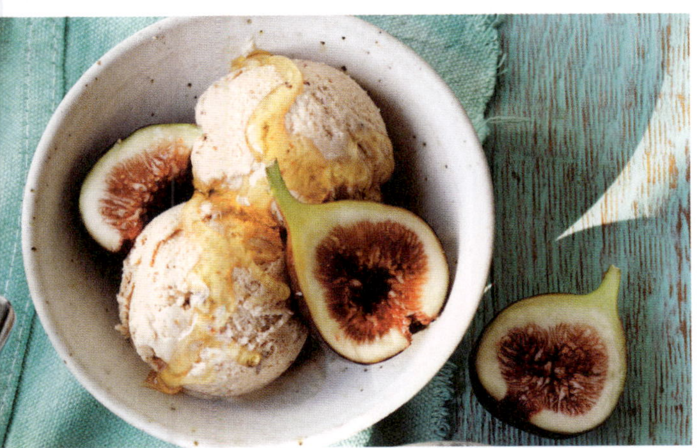

Contents

Mediterranean Life

The Mediterranean diet is an approach to healthy eating that embraces variety, flavor, and nutrient-rich foods. Often referred to as the world's healthiest diet, it's backed by an abundance of scientific evidence showing that people who eat the Mediterranean way live longer and healthier lives.

Why eat the Mediterranean way?

It's no secret that people who eat a Mediterranean diet share many commonalities, including a longer life expectancy, healthier hearts, and lower rates of chronic disease. The positive effects of the diet are far reaching and include lower levels of "bad" LDL cholesterol, better blood glucose (sugar) control, improved weight management, reduced risk of depression, and a lower incidence of some cancers as well as Parkinson's and Alzheimer's diseases.

The Mediterranean diet is centered on minimally processed foods such as whole grains, fruits, and vegetables, as well as seafood and fish, yogurt, legumes, seeds, and nuts. Also included are many foods often seen as indulgences, such as red wine, olive oil, butter, and bread—because, ultimately, balance and enjoyment are the core of this lifestyle.

Healthy fats

When it comes to good nutrition, not all fats are created equal, but cutting out fat isn't encouraged in a Mediterranean diet. In fact, including healthy fats as part of a balanced diet can actually promote better health and may be the reason why people who follow a Mediterranean diet have healthier hearts than those who eat a traditional Western diet.

Healthy fats, including olive oil, nuts and seeds, oily fish, and dairy products like yogurt are all included on the Mediterranean menu. Olive oil is the primary source of fat—it's an excellent source of monounsaturated fat and linoleic acid, both of which are good news for your heart. Note that "extra virgin" and "virgin" oil are the least processed options while also containing the highest levels of beneficial polyphenols—the protective antioxidant phytochemical compounds found in plants.

With the Mediterranean diet you simply swap sources of saturated and trans fats for foods with more monounsaturated and polyunsaturated fats. Choose foods like avocado, nuts, seeds, oily fish, extra virgin olive oil, and dairy products rather than filling up on too much red meat or deep-fried and processed options.

Ocean catch

Seafood and fish are at the heart of this diet, offering a healthier and more sustainable alternative to red meat. Oily fish, such as sardines, herring tuna, salmon, and mackerel, are all good sources of heart-healthy omega-3 fatty acids, a polyunsaturated fat that can help boost brain function, including memory, concentration, and mood. Eat fish or seafood at least twice a week and stick to smaller portions of red meat no more than two or three times a week. Along with seafood, plant-based sources of protein, such as legumes, nuts, and seeds, are heavily emphasized in the Mediterranean kitchen, making sure the body receives key nutrition.

Fiber-rich foods

The Mediterranean diet also includes plenty of unrefined whole grains and other fiber-rich foods such as vegetables and fruit to fuel your body with naturally slow-burning energy sources. A diet high in fiber is linked to better weight management and digestion, more stable mood, improved cholesterol levels, and reduced risk of some diseases, including bowel cancer. Choose whole grains such as oats, brown and black rice, quinoa, freekeh, and barley over the more refined and processed options. Adding legumes into your diet is also a great way to up your fiber intake and stay fuller for longer.

Many Mediterranean dishes are naturally bright and colorful, thanks to the fresh, seasonal produce that is key to creating such delicious, balanced meals. Fruit and vegetables are naturally full of antioxidants and polyphenols, which help combat signs of aging and reduce the risk of inflammatory diseases. Eat five to ten portions of vegetables and fruit a day to get plenty of health-boosting antioxidants, polyphenols, vitamins, minerals, and fiber into your diet.

The Mediterranean lifestyle

It's not just the sorts of foods consumed in the Mediterranean diet that makes it so good for you, it's the way in which the food is cooked and eaten, with importance placed on fresh, quality produce, mealtimes, and balanced portion sizes.

Most Mediterranean dishes are designed to be enjoyed with family and friends, and this communal approach to eating helps to develop a sense of community and connection that is essential to well-being and happiness. Sharing dishes around the table also helps foster a healthy relationship with food, where the focus is on enjoyment and satiation rather than on restriction or control. Eating at the table is just one simple step that can promote mindfulness at mealtimes.

Another benefit of eating family-style shared plates is that it encourages variety, which is the core of the Mediterranean diet. Including a wide range of ingredients in an array of colors is a simple way to help your body get a healthy mix of everything it needs to work its best—choose mostly plant foods and try new ingredients, particularly as the seasons change. As you fill up on more nutrient-rich foods, you'll help your body thrive.

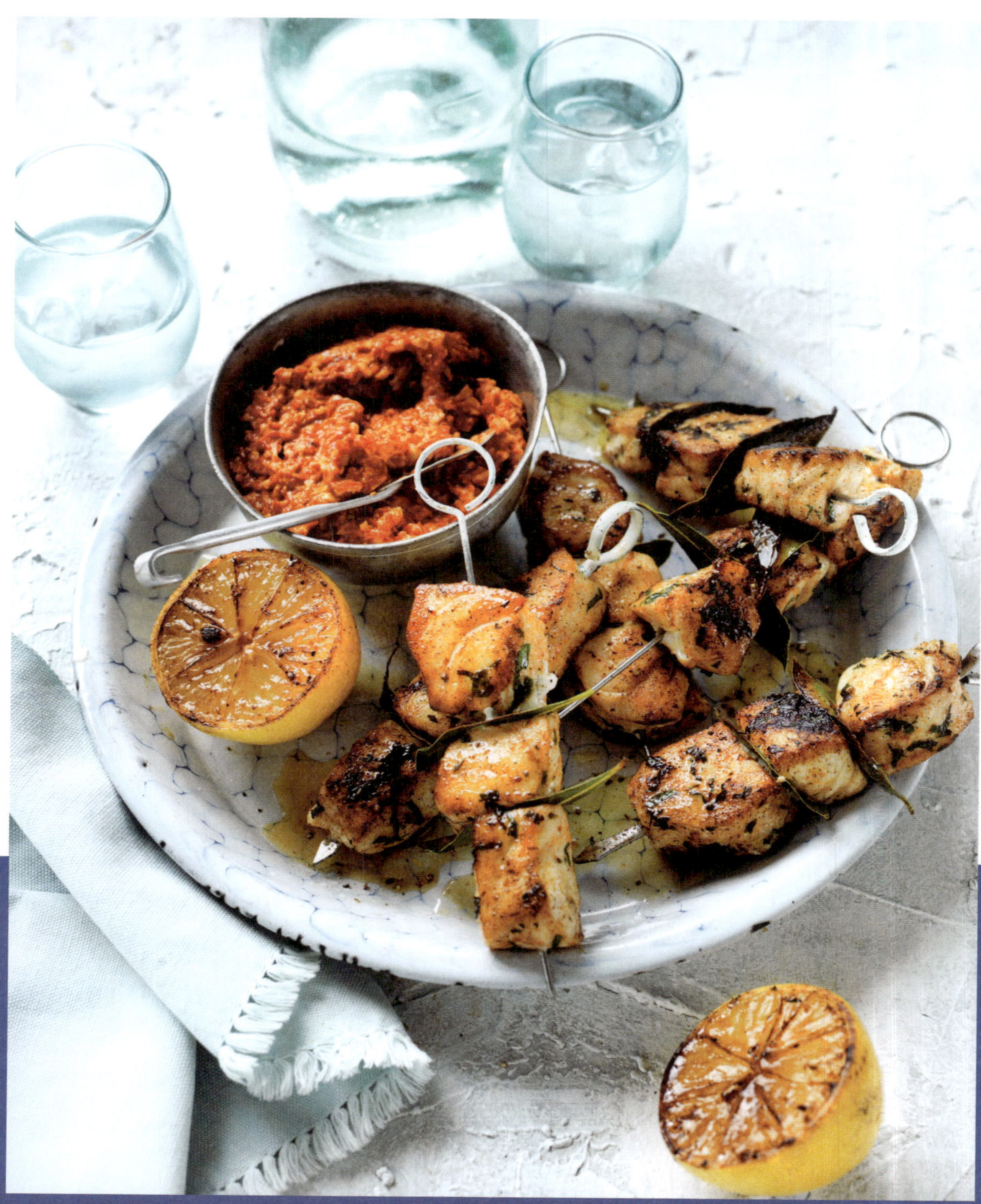

SHARED PLATES

From starters to tapas and light bites, these dishes will add vibrancy to your table. Perfect for sharing, they'll bring a sense of communal enjoyment to group gatherings.

Spring greens and feta bruschetta

VEGETARIAN | PREP + COOK TIME **40 MINUTES** | SERVES **4**

Pesto alla genovese is a sauce originating in Genoa, Italy. It is traditionally made by pounding or grinding garlic cloves, pine nuts, basil, cheese, and olive oil together using a mortar and pestle. Today there are many variations of pesto, from this one, with arugula and almonds, to others that use different fresh green herbs or even spinach or kale.

1 cup frozen fava beans, thawed (see tips)
1/3lb (170g) asparagus, trimmed, sliced diagonally
1/2 cup frozen peas
8 slices sourdough bread
2 tbsp olive oil, divided
1 garlic clove, crushed
1 tbsp lemon juice
salt and freshly ground black pepper
3oz (90g) drained marinated feta cheese, crumbled
2 tbsp small fresh mint leaves
1 tsp finely grated lemon zest

arugula and almond pesto

3 cups arugula
1 cup fresh basil leaves
1/2 cup slivered almonds, roasted
1 garlic clove, crushed
1 tsp finely grated lemon zest
1/3 cup finely grated Parmesan cheese
1/2 cup olive oil

1 Cook the fava beans and asparagus in a medium saucepan of boiling water for 2 minutes. Add the peas, cook for 2 minutes; drain. Plunge in a bowl of ice water; drain. Remove gray skins from the fava beans. Set aside.

2 To make the arugula and almond pesto, combine the arugula, basil, almonds, garlic, lemon zest, Parmesan cheese, and 1 tbsp of the olive oil in a food processor and pulse until coarsely chopped. With the processor running, add the remaining oil in a thin, steady stream until the mixture is smooth; season with salt and pepper to taste.

3 Brush each side of the bread with 1 tbsp of the olive oil. Cook the bread on a heated grill (barbecue) or ridged grill pan for 1 minute on each side or until lightly charred. Spread 1/3 cup of pesto on the bread slices.

4 Heat the remaining olive oil in a medium frying pan over medium-high heat. Cook the garlic for 1 minute. Add the asparagus, beans, and peas; cook for 2–3 minutes or until hot. Stir in the lemon juice; season with salt and pepper to taste.

5 Spoon the vegetable mixture onto the toasted bread; top with the feta cheese, mint, and lemon zest.

TIPS

- If fresh fava beans are in season, you may use 1 1/4lb (575g) fresh fava beans instead of frozen. Simply shell and cook them in the same way.
- Serving-sized portions of pesto can be frozen in small tightly sealed containers for up to 3 months.

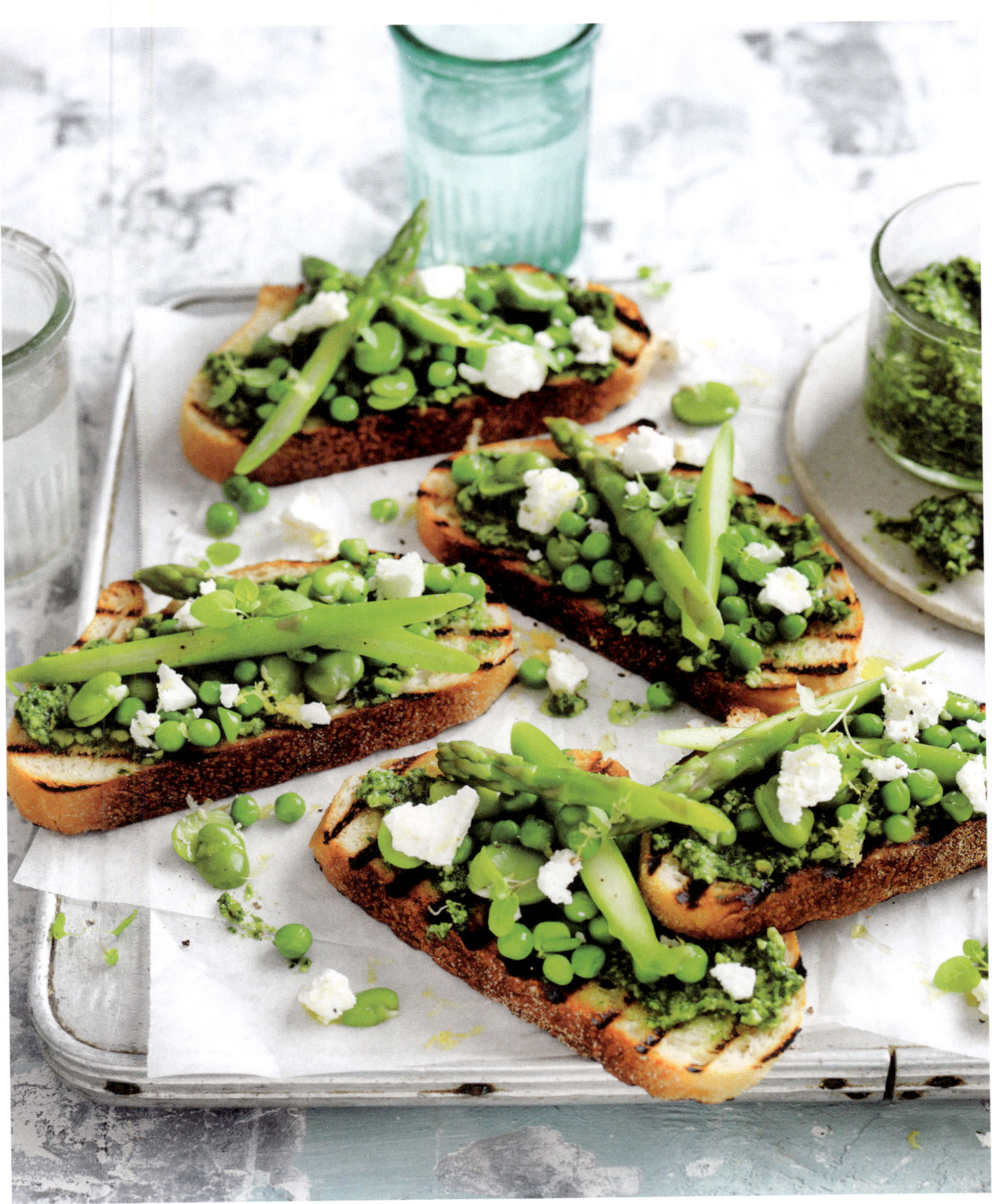

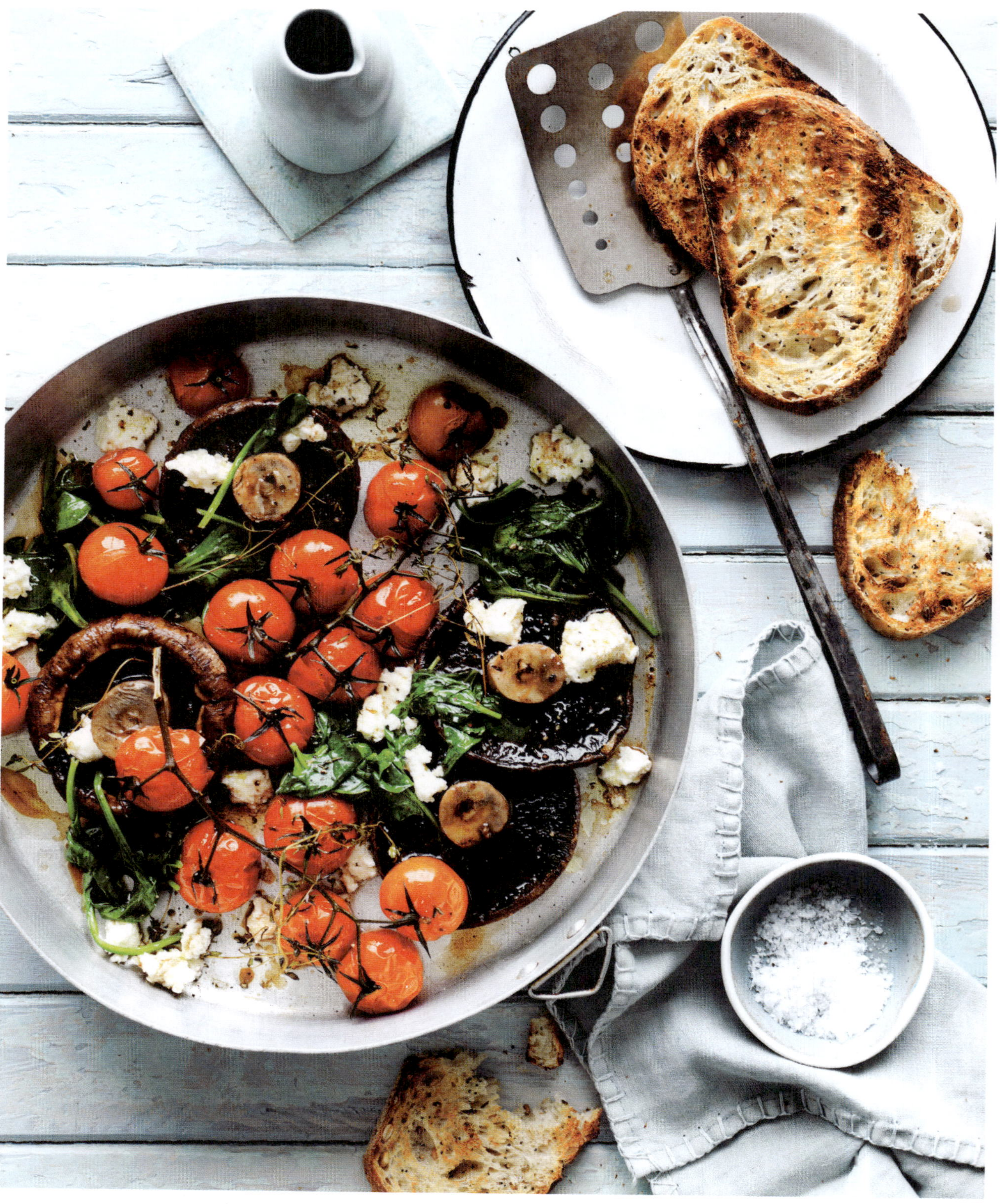

Roasted mushrooms with spinach, tomato, and ricotta cheese

VEGETARIAN | PREP + COOK TIME **40 MINUTES** | SERVES **2**

Soft, sweet, moist ricotta cheese is made from cow's milk, with a low fat content and a slightly grainy texture. The name roughly translates as "cooked again" and refers to the cheese's manufacture from a whey that is itself a by-product of other cheese making. Ricotta cheese has been made in Italy for centuries and has a special place in Italian cuisine.

4 large portobello mushrooms
10oz (275g) cherry tomatoes
2 tbsp olive oil, divided
salt and freshly ground black pepper
2 garlic cloves, crushed
1 tbsp balsamic vinegar
12 sprigs fresh thyme
1½ cups (50g) baby spinach leaves
¼ cup fresh ricotta, crumbled
sourdough bread slices, toasted, for serving

1. Preheat the oven to 400°F (200°C). Line a large baking sheet with parchment paper.
2. Place the mushrooms and tomatoes on the lined baking sheet; drizzle evenly with 1 tbsp of olive oil. Season with salt and pepper.
3. Combine the garlic, vinegar, and remaining olive oil in a small bowl; drizzle over the mushrooms, then sprinkle with the thyme. Cover the pan loosely with parchment paper; bake for 20 minutes.
4. Discard the parchment paper cover. Tuck the spinach leaves under the mushrooms and tomatoes. Top the mushrooms with the ricotta cheese. Bake for 5 minutes or until vegetables are tender. Serve with toasted sourdough.

TIP

In many supermarkets, portobello mushrooms are sold simply as large mushroom caps suitable for stuffing. They work beautifully in this recipe.

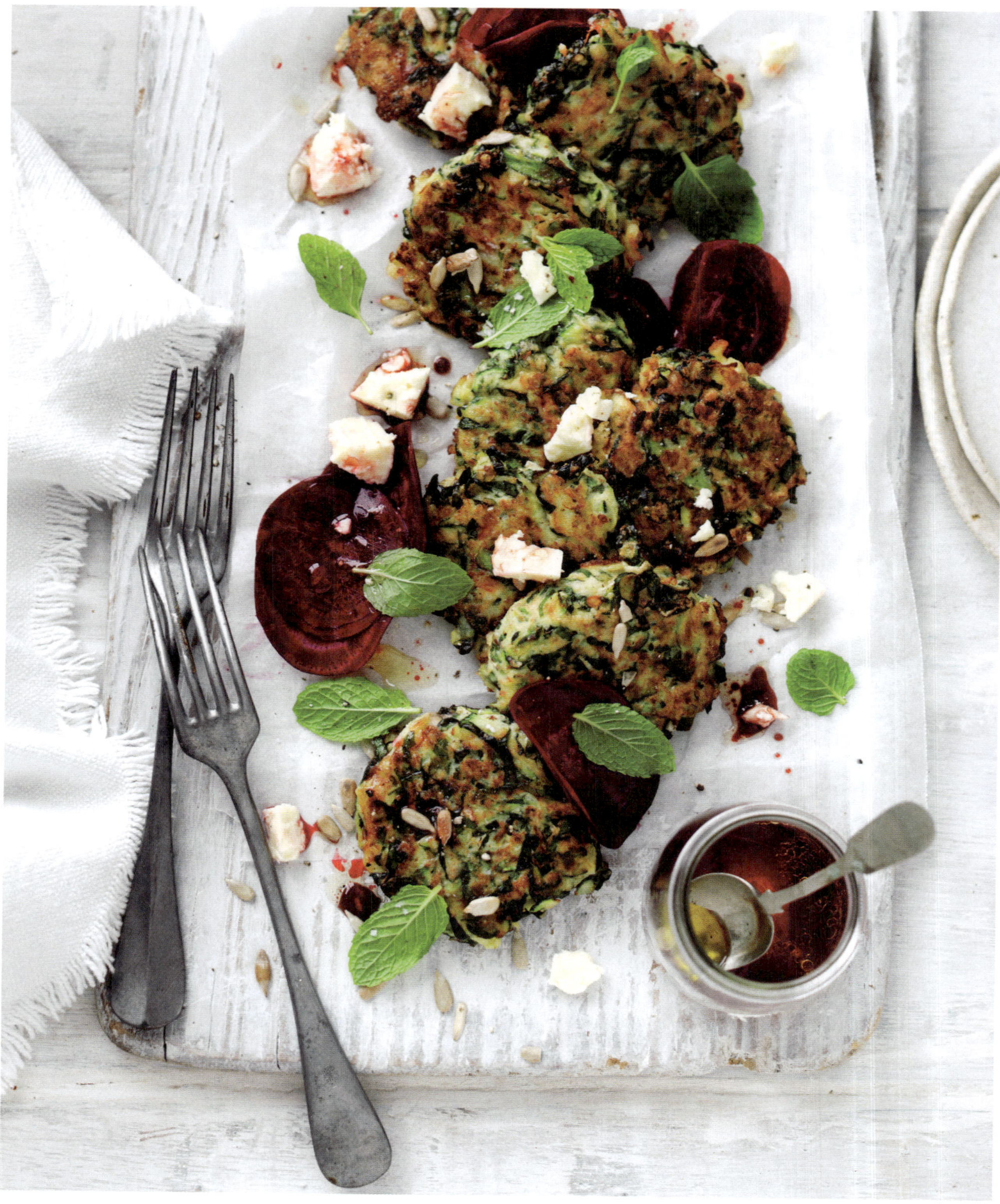

Tuscan kale fritters with pickled beets

VEGETARIAN | PREP + COOK TIME **35 MINUTES + STANDING** | SERVES **4**

Tuscan kale, also known as cavolo nero or "black cabbage" in Italian, is featured in many Italian dishes, especially those from Tuscany. The traditional ingredient of minestrone soup, Tuscan kale is more delicate and sweet than its relative, curly kale, but possesses many of the same nutritional benefits; it is rich in protein, fiber, antioxidants, and vitamins.

3 large zucchini, coarsely grated
1 tsp fine sea salt
3 Tuscan kale (or any variety) leaves, trimmed, finely shredded
2 tbsp chopped fresh mint leaves
1/4 cup whole wheat flour
2 garlic cloves, crushed
2 eggs, lightly beaten
salt and freshly ground black pepper
1/3 cup olive oil, divided
1 tbsp apple cider vinegar
1/2 tsp honey
4oz (100g) feta cheese, crumbled
2 tbsp sunflower seeds, toasted
fresh mint leaves, to garnish

pickled beets
3 small beets, peeled, thinly sliced (see tips)
2 tbsp apple cider vinegar

1. Combine the zucchini and salt in a strainer over a bowl for 10 minutes to drain. Using your hands, squeeze excess liquid from the zucchini. Place the zucchini, kale, mint, flour, garlic, and egg in a medium bowl; season with salt and pepper. Mix well to combine.
2. Meanwhile, make the pickled beets. Combine the beets and vinegar in a bowl; season with salt and pepper. Let stand for 5–15 minutes. Drain, reserving the pickling liquid for the honey dressing. Set aside.
3. Heat 2 tbsp of the olive oil in a large nonstick frying pan over medium heat. Add an eighth of the zucchini and kale mixture to the pan, flatten slightly; cook for 5 minutes on each side or until golden and crisp. Drain on paper towel; cover to keep warm. Repeat with the remaining mixture to make eight fritters.
4. Make the honey dressing. Whisk the remaining oil, vinegar, honey, and reserved pickling liquid in a small bowl until combined.
5. Place the fritters on a platter, top with the pickled beets and feta cheese. Before serving, drizzle with the honey dressing and sprinkle with the sunflower seeds and mint leaves.

TIPS

- You can use a mandoline or V-slicer to slice the beet very thinly.
- Cooked fritters can be frozen; reheat for a quick breakfast option.

Sardine and yellow tomato toasts

PESCATARIAN | PREP + COOK TIME **30 MINUTES + REFRIGERATION** | SERVES **4**

Fresh sardines are not in season for very long in the US, so when they become available it's worth it to catch a few at your fishmongers. If you can't find any, try Spanish mackerel for a full-flavored fish substitute. You can also substitute high-quality sardine filets packed in a jar. These are available through your local gourmet store or online.

1 tsp fennel seeds, lightly crushed
2 tsp sea salt flakes
2 garlic cloves, finely chopped
salt and freshly ground black pepper
1lb (500g) fresh sardines, cleaned, filleted, with tails intact (see tip)
10oz (285g) yellow cherry tomatoes
1/4 cup olive oil, divided
1 loaf ciabatta bread, sliced, toasted
small fresh basil leaves, to garnish
lemon wedges, for serving

basil and caperberry oil

1 cup fresh basil leaves
1/2 cup olive oil
1/4 cup caperberries
2 tsp finely grated lemon zest
2 tbsp lemon juice

1 Combine all the ingredients for the basil and caperberry oil in a food processor and pulse until smooth; season with salt and pepper to taste. Set aside.

2 In a small bowl, combine the fennel seeds, salt, and garlic; season with salt and pepper. Rub this fennel mixture over the sardine fillets. Cover; refrigerate for 30 minutes.

3 Preheat the oven to 500°F (250°C) or turn the broiler on high. On a baking sheet, add the tomatoes and coat them in 4 tbsp of the olive oil. Bake or broil for 10 minutes or until the tomatoes are just starting to blister. Cool slightly.

4 Place the tomatoes, the basil, and the caperberry oil in a large bowl; toss gently to combine. Season with salt and pepper to taste.

5 Heat the remaining oil in a large sauté pan or preheat a ridged grill pan without oil. If using a grill pan, rub the fish in oil. Cook the sardines, in batches, for 2 minutes on each side or until cooked.

6 Place the sardines on the toasted bread; spoon the tomato mixture on top, pressing gently to allow tomato juices to soak into the bread. Top with the basil leaves; serve with lemon wedges.

TIPS

- Ask the fishmonger to clean and fillet the sardines.
- Caperberries are packed in brine in a jar; you'll find them in the grocery store near the olives and capers.

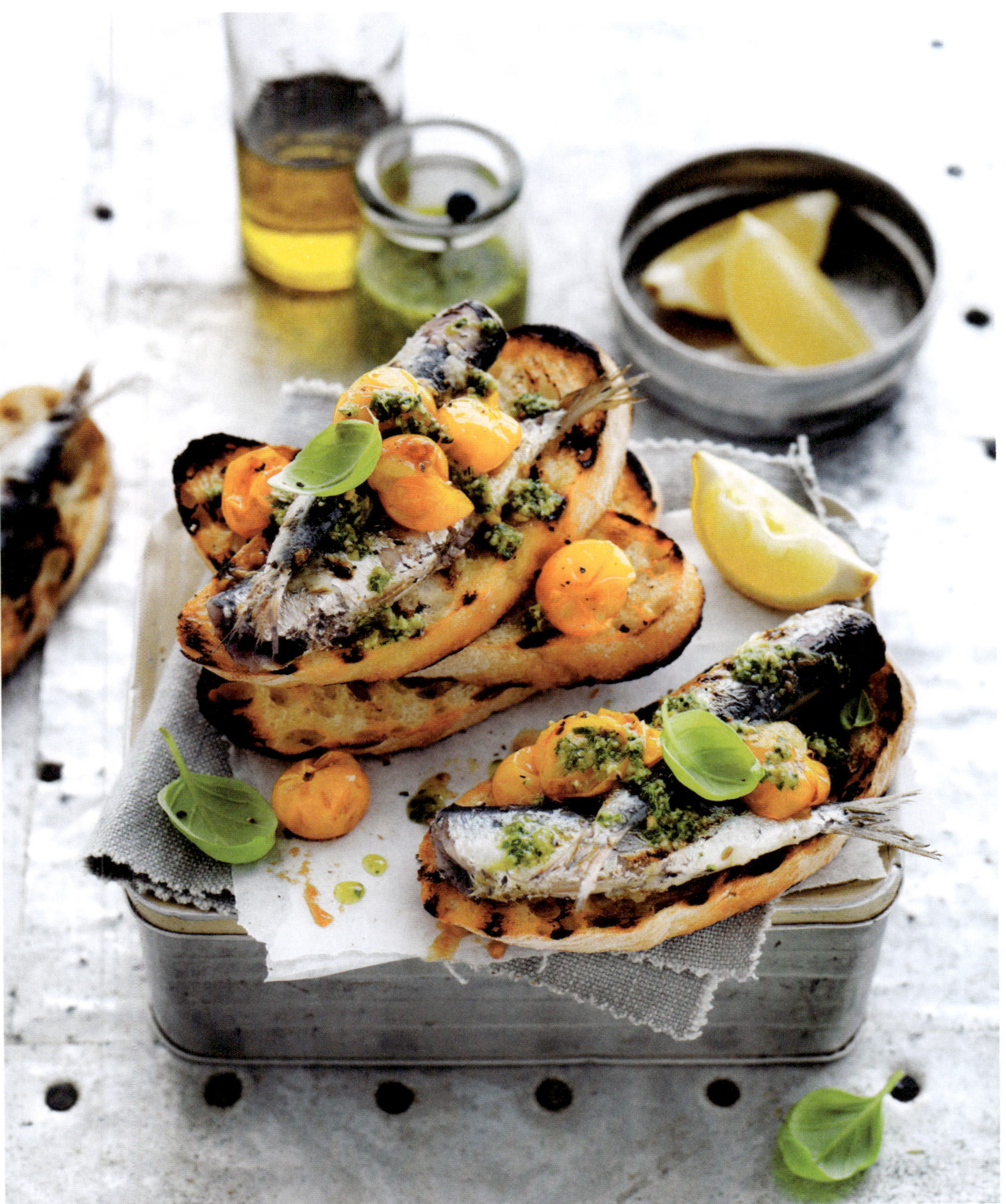

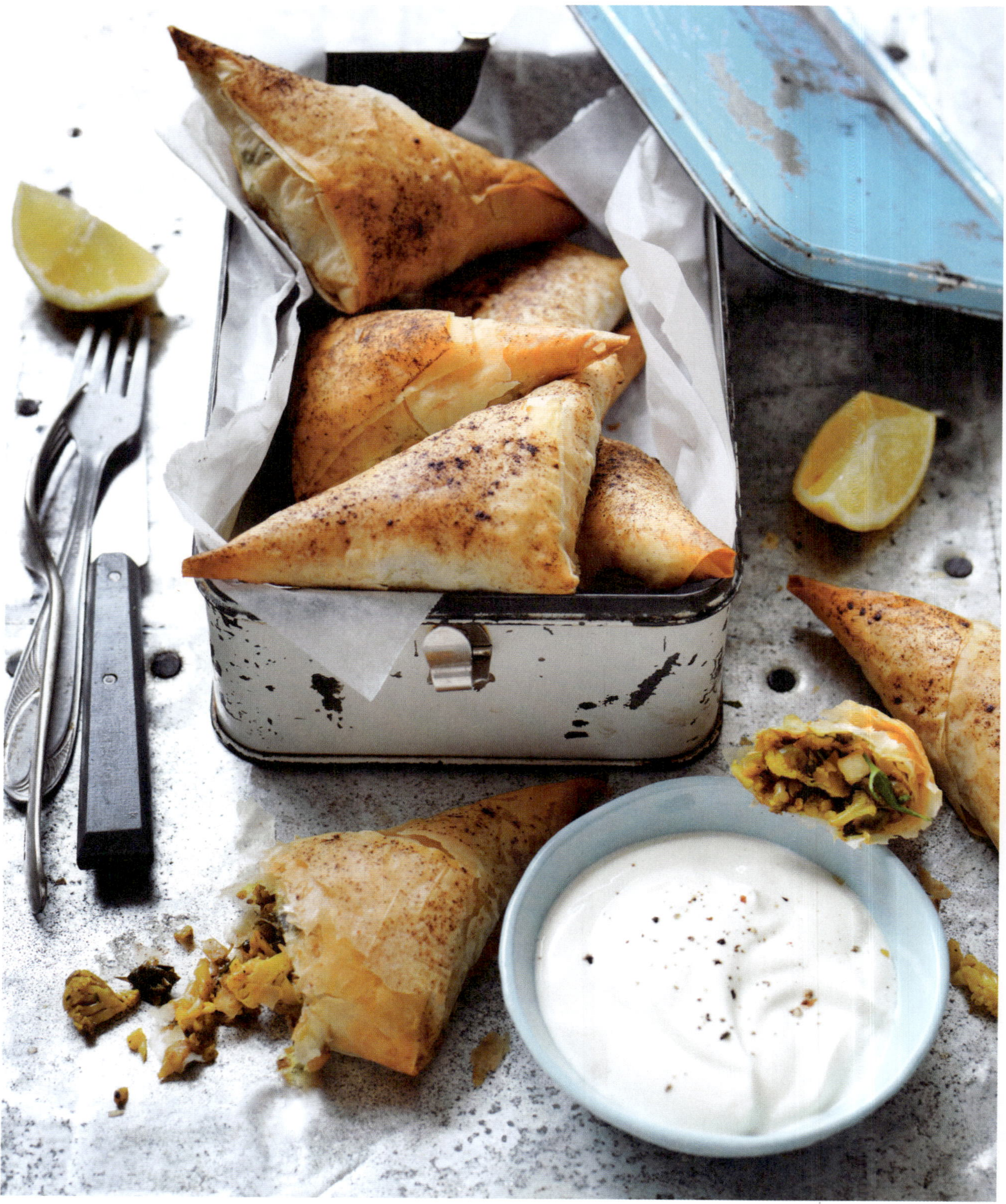

Cauliflower pastilla triangles

VEGAN | PREP + COOK TIME **1 HOUR 20 MINUTES + STANDING** | MAKES **9**

Pastilla is a traditional Moroccan pie served on special occasions. Although usually filled with a lightly spiced mix of poultry and nuts, this vegan version instead stars cauliflower. Saffron is one of the most expensive spices in the world by weight—it consists of the dried stigmas of the crocus plant, and a kilogram of saffron requires 110,000–170,000 flowers.

pinch of saffron threads
1/2 cup plus 2 tbsp oil
2 medium red onions (about 1 1/2 cups), finely chopped
2 garlic cloves, crushed
1 tsp ground turmeric
1 tsp ground ginger
3/4 tsp ground cinnamon, divided
1 medium head cauliflower (about 2 cups of florets), finely chopped
salt
1 cup roasted blanched almonds, roughly chopped
1 cup fresh cilantro leaves, roughly chopped
1 cup fresh Italian parsley leaves, roughly chopped
9 sheets phyllo pastry, 14 x 18 in (36 x 46cm)
lemon wedges, for serving
Greek yogurt, for serving

1 Combine the saffron and 1 tbsp hot water in a small bowl.

2 Heat 2 tbsp olive oil in a large skillet over medium heat; cook the onion, garlic, turmeric, ginger, and 1/2 tsp of the ground cinnamon for 5 minutes or until the onion softens. Add the cauliflower; cook, stirring, for 10 minutes or until tender. Season with salt. Add the saffron mixture; cook for 1 minute or until the water evaporates. Transfer to a large bowl; stir in the almonds and herbs. Let cool completely.

3 Preheat oven to 350°F (180°C). Line a large baking sheet with parchment paper.

4 Brush one sheet of pastry with a little of the remaining oil; cut in half lengthwise, place one strip directly on top of the other. Keep the remaining sheets covered with parchment paper topped with a clean, damp kitchen towel to prevent them from drying out.

5 Place about 1/2 cup of the cauliflower mixture in a corner of the pastry strip, leaving a 1/2in (1cm) border. Fold the opposite corner of the pastry diagonally across the filling to form a triangle; continue folding to the end of the pastry sheet, retaining the triangular shape. Brush on a small amount of water to seal the pastry, if needed. Place the triangle, seam-side down, on the baking sheet. Repeat with the remaining pastry, oil, and cauliflower filling.

6 Brush the triangles with a little more oil; dust with the remaining cinnamon. Bake for 30 minutes or until the pastry is lightly browned.

7 Serve warm with lemon wedges and Greek yogurt, if desired.

Small bites

Tapas—small plates or appetizers—originate from Spain, but every Mediterranean country has its own versions. Great for serving at parties, these bites can be enjoyed as a snack or appetizer, or combined to create a full sharing meal.

Dukkah shrimp skewers

PESCATARIAN | PREP TIME **15 MINUTES** | SERVES **4**

Peel and devein 2½lb (1.2kg) uncooked large shrimp, leaving the tails intact. Combine ¼ cup pistachio dukkah, 2 tbsp of olive oil, 2 crushed garlic cloves, and 2 tsp of finely grated lemon zest in a large bowl; add the shrimp, toss to coat in mixture. Thread shrimp onto 8 metal or soaked bamboo skewers. Heat a ridged grill pan or heavy sauté pan over high heat; cook the skewers, turning, until shrimp change color. Serve with lemon wedges.

Baked feta cheese with roasted garlic, chile, and olives

VEGETARIAN | PREP TIME **1 HOUR 25 MINUTES** | SERVES **10**

Preheat oven to 350°F (180°C). Place 10 unpeeled cloves of garlic and ¼ cup olive oil in a small baking dish. Cover with foil; bake for 30 minutes or until tender. Let cool slightly. Slip roasted cloves out of their peels. Set aside. Reserve any remaining oil. Increase oven to 400°F (200°C). Pat a 10oz (300g) block of feta cheese dry with paper towel. Cut into 1½in (4cm) thick slices; place in a baking dish just large enough for feta cheese to fit in a single layer. Pour ¼ cup additional olive oil and add garlic and its oil over the feta cheese; top with 2 sprigs fresh rosemary, 3 tsp of fresh oregano leaves, ⅓ cup small black olives, and half of a thinly sliced fresh long red chile. Bake for 40 minutes or until the feta cheese is soft and lightly browned. Serve with toasted or grilled pita bread.

Stuffed zucchini flowers

VEGETARIAN | PREP TIME **2 HOURS 30 MINUTES** | MAKES **18**

Combine 1 cup firm ricotta cheese, ¼ cup crumbled feta cheese, 2 tbsp of finely chopped fresh mint leaves, 2 tsp of finely grated lemon zest, ½ tsp of dried chile flakes, 1 crushed garlic clove, and 1 egg yolk in a medium bowl; season with salt and pepper to taste. Carefully open 18 zucchini flowers then remove the yellow stamens from inside the flowers. Gently spoon the ricotta cheese mixture into the flowers, leaving a ½in (1cm) gap at the top. Twist the petal tops to enclose the filling. Heat 2 tbsp of olive oil in a nonstick sauté pan over high heat; cook the flowers for 1 minute on each side or until slightly golden and heated through; season with salt and pepper to taste. Sprinkle with finely grated lemon zest and mint leaves.

CLOCKWISE from top

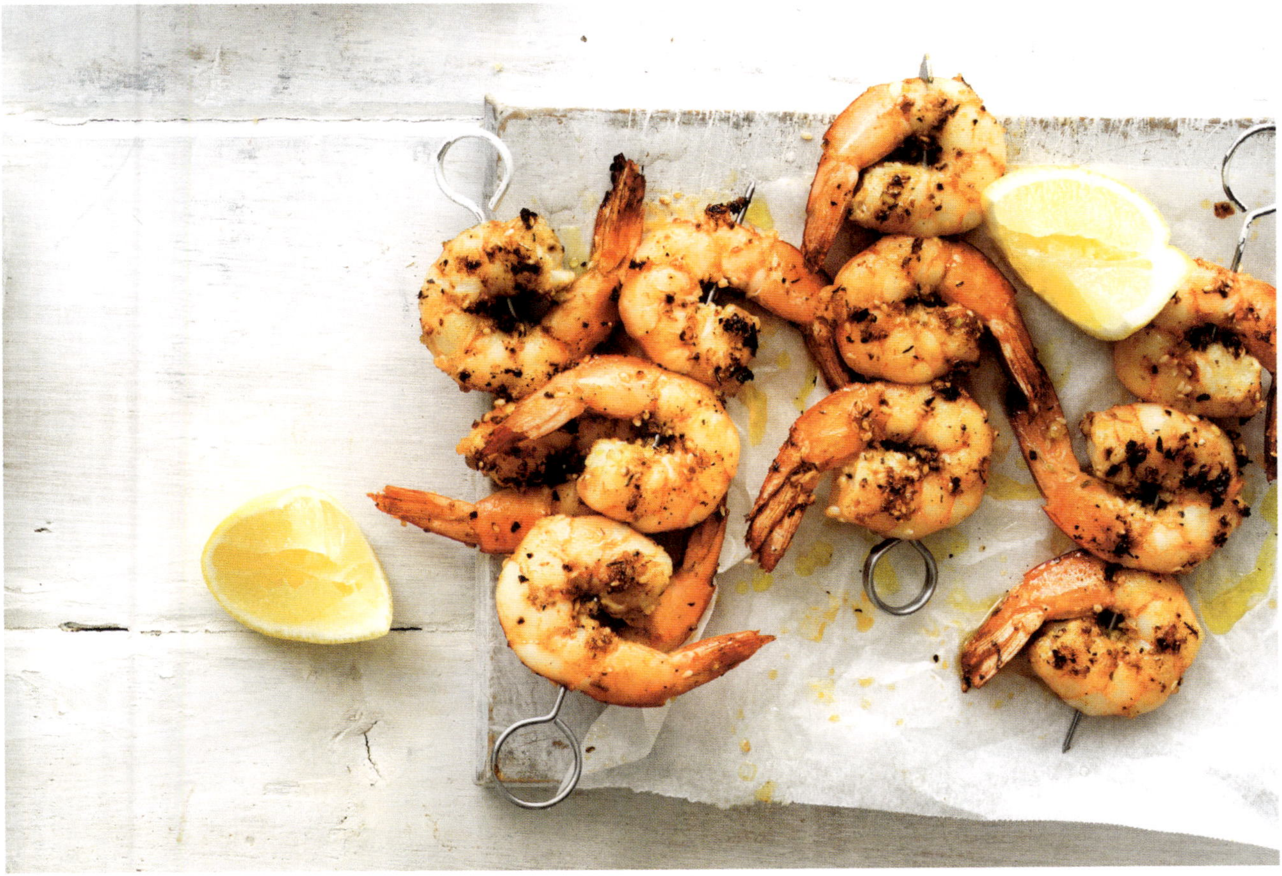

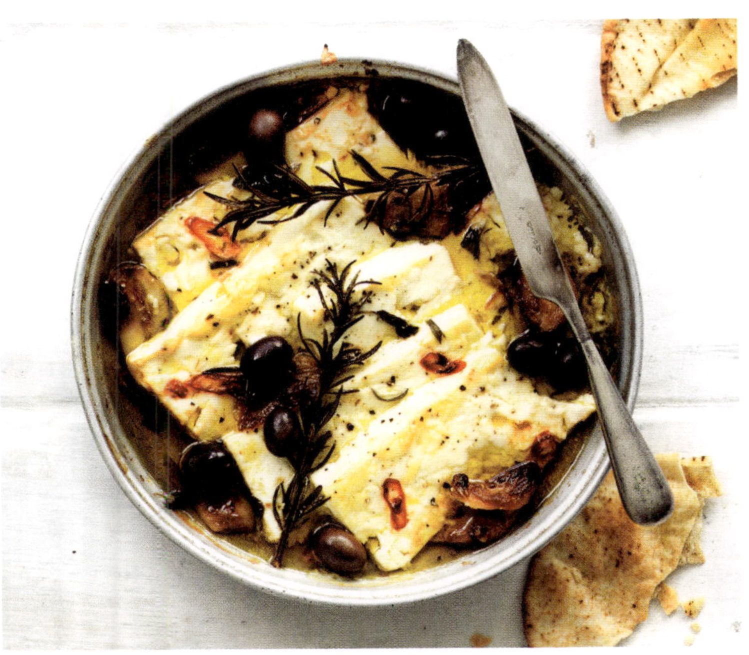

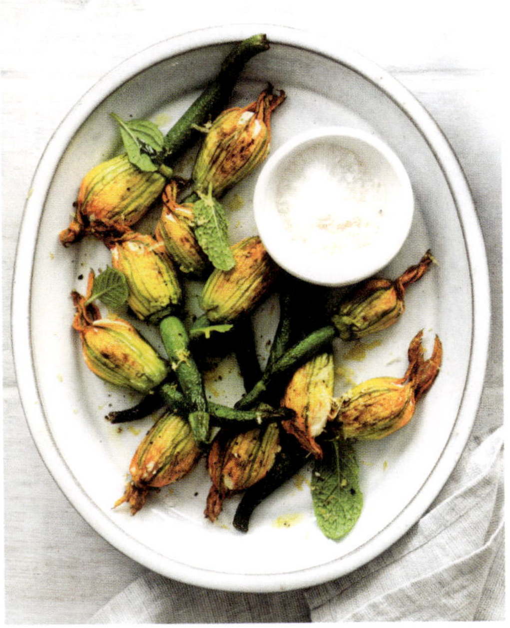

Grilled sardines with pangrattato

PESCATARIAN | PREP + COOK TIME **20 MINUTES** | SERVES **4**

Pangrattato is Italian for breadcrumbs. In southern parts of the country this crunchy topping was used as a substitute for more expensive cheese. Recently, seasoned breadcrumbs have become popular as a delicious topping for vegetables, salads, and pasta, and they're great sprinkled on crispy fried eggs. It's a perfect way to use up old, stale bread and save it from the trash.

1½lb (750g) fresh sardines, cleaned (see tips)
¼ cup olive oil, divided, plus extra to serve
salt and freshly ground black pepper
1 medium lemon
1¾oz arugula
⅓ cup watercress (see tips)
¼ cup pine nuts, toasted (see tips)

pangrattato
2 tbsp olive oil
1 cup day-old bread, roughly chopped
1 garlic clove, crushed
½ cup fresh Italian parsley, roughly chopped
¼ cup finely grated Parmesan cheese

1. To make the pangrattato, heat the olive oil in a large frying pan over medium heat; cook the bread, stirring, for 2 minutes or until golden. Add the garlic; cook, stirring, for 1 minute or until fragrant. Let cool for 10 minutes. In a food processor, add the bread and parsley; pulse until coarse crumbs form. Stir in the Parmesan cheese; season with salt and pepper to taste.
2. Rub the sardines with 2 tbsp of olive oil; season with salt and pepper. Cook the sardines on a heated grill (barbecue) or ridged grill pan over high heat for 2 minutes. Turn, cook for 1 minute or until cooked through.
3. Cut the lemon in half; juice one half, cut the remaining half into wedges. Place the arugula, watercress, pine nuts, lemon juice, and remaining oil in a medium bowl. Season with salt and pepper.
4. Place the arugula mixture on a platter; top with the sardines, then drizzle with a little more olive oil. Sprinkle with the pangrattato. Serve with the lemon wedges.

TIPS

- Ask the fishmonger to clean the sardines. If you can't find fresh sardines, substitute Spanish mackerel or sardine filets packed in a jar.
- Substitute any salad leaves for watercress.
- Substitute your favorite toasted nuts or seeds for the pine nuts.

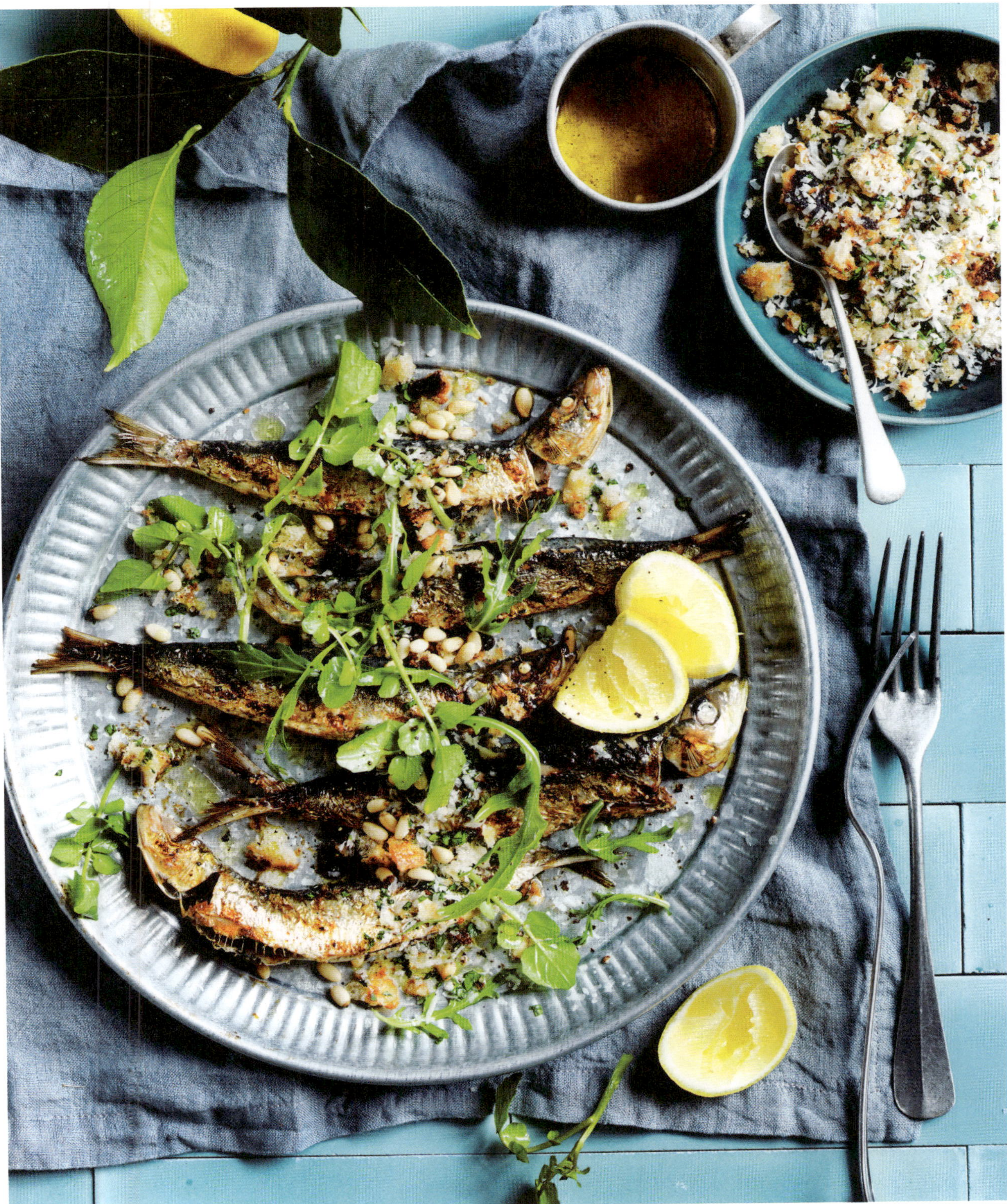

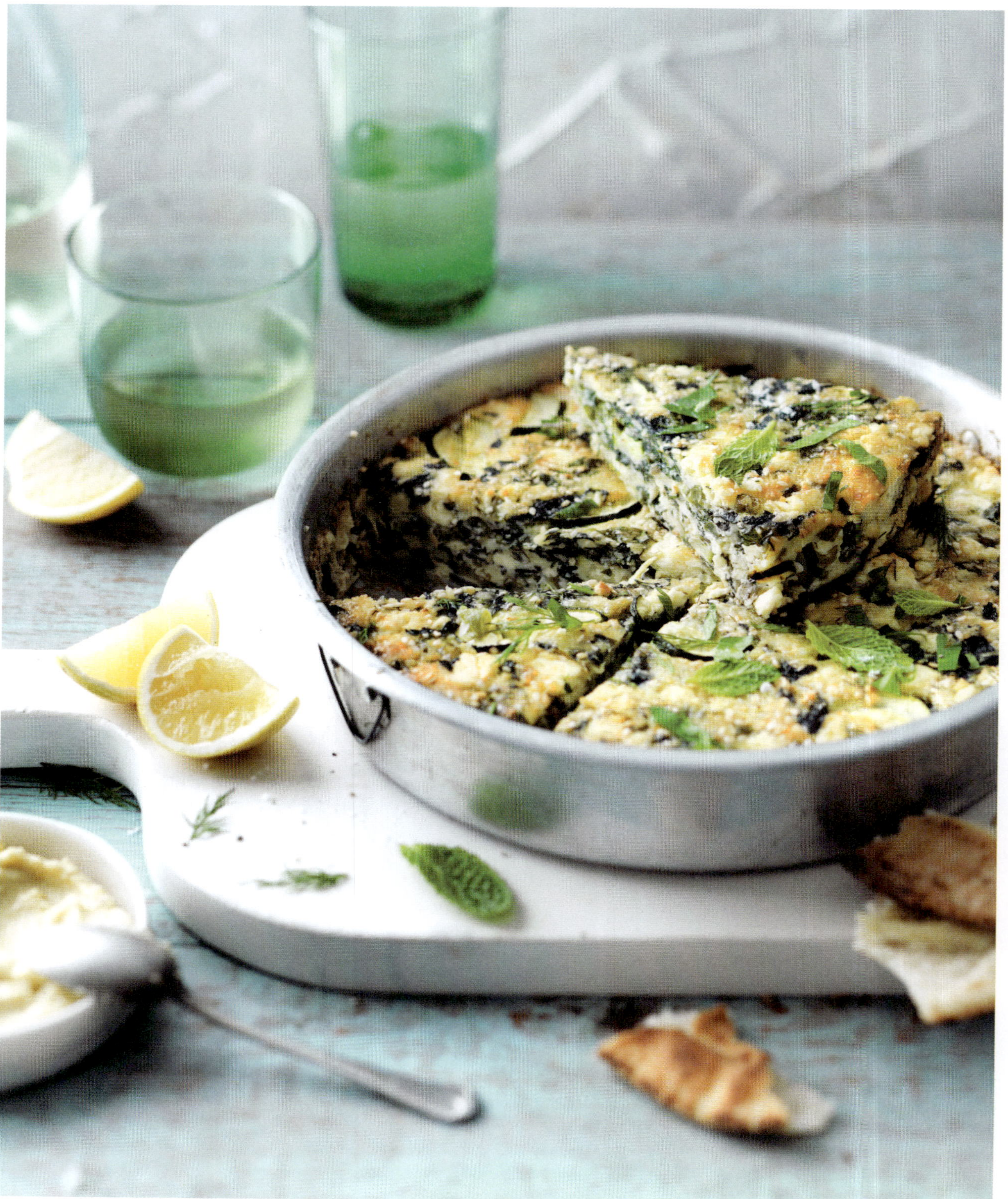

Greek vegetable pie with yellow split pea dip

VEGETARIAN | PREP + COOK TIME **1 HOUR 15 MINUTES + STANDING & COOLING** | SERVES **8**

Although it's called a pie, this traditional Greek baked vegetable-and-herb-packed recipe is more like a frittata because it contains no pastry. You can boost the flavor by sprinkling it with fresh small mint leaves before serving, if you like.

2 medium zucchini, very thinly sliced
1 tsp fine sea salt
1 bunch Swiss chard, thinly sliced (about 3 cups)
½ lb (225g) fresh green beans, trimmed
½ cup feta cheese, crumbled
½ cup Parmigiano-Reggiano cheese, grated
¼ cup fresh Italian parsley leaves, roughly chopped
2 tbsp chopped fresh dill
1 tbsp chopped fresh mint leaves
¾ cup fresh breadcrumbs (see tips)
6 eggs, lightly beaten
¼ cup sesame seeds, toasted
1 tbsp olive oil
salt and freshly ground black pepper
8 small pita breads, warmed
lemon wedges, for serving

yellow split pea dip

1 cup dried yellow split peas
1 small onion, chopped
4 garlic cloves, bruised
1 tsp ground cumin
1 tsp ground coriander
⅓ cup olive oil
¼ cup lemon juice

TIP

The breadcrumbs are best made from bread that is about 3 days old.

1 Preheat the oven to 350°F (180°C). Coat the inside of a 9in (23cm) springform pan with cooking spray; cut a circle from parchment paper to fit the bottom. Wrap the outside bottom of the pan in aluminum foil.

2 Combine the zucchini and salt in a strainer over a bowl; let stand for 30 minutes. Rinse the zucchini under cold water; drain. Meanwhile, trim stems from the Swiss chard; discard stems.

3 Meanwhile, cook the green beans in a large saucepan of boiling water for 5 minutes or until crisp tender. Remove and finely chop the beans.

4 Add the chard to the water in the pan, return to a boil; drain immediately. Cool under cold running water; drain well. Squeeze to remove excess moisture; pat dry with paper towel. Finely chop the wilted chard leaves.

5 Place the zucchini, green beans, and chard in a large bowl with the cheeses, herbs, breadcrumbs, egg, sesame seeds, and olive oil; mix well to combine. Season with salt and pepper. Spoon the mixture into the springform pan; smooth the surface.

6 Bake the pie for 35 minutes or until golden and set. Leave in the pan for 15 minutes.

7 Meanwhile, to make the yellow split pea dip, place the split peas in a small saucepan with enough cold water to just cover; bring to a boil for just a few minutes, then drain, rinse. Return the peas to the pan with the onion and garlic, add enough cold water to cover by 2¼in (6cm); bring to a boil. Reduce heat to medium; cook for 25 minutes or until the peas are tender and beginning to collapse. Drain. Cool to room temperature.

8 In a food processor, add the split pea mixture and spices. Pulse until smooth. With the processor running, gradually add the olive oil in a steady stream, then add the lemon juice in a steady stream. Season with salt and pepper to taste.

9 Serve pie warm or room temperature with dip, pita, and lemon wedges.

Whole-wheat pizza marinara

PESCATARIAN | PREP + COOK TIME **45 MINUTES + REFRIGERATION AND STANDING** | SERVES **4**

This healthy substitute for takeout pizza ditches the greasy calorie-laden cheese for low-fat seafood chile marinara on a crispy whole wheat crust. Your fishmonger can clean the octopus for you, but many supermarkets and international groceries sell fresh or frozen packaged octopus, which is just as easy to use.

8 uncooked medium-sized shrimp
3/4 lbs (360g) fresh or frozen octopus, cut into large pieces
2 fresh long red chiles, finely chopped
2 garlic cloves, crushed
2 tsp finely grated lemon zest
2 tbsp olive oil
salt and freshly ground black pepper
10oz (285g) cherry tomatoes, halved
1 1/2 cups arugula
1 tbsp lemon juice
lemon wedges, to serve

dough

1/4 cup bulgur
1/2 tsp sugar
1 tsp dry yeast
2/3 cup all-purpose flour
2/3 cup whole wheat flour

1 Peel and devein the shrimp; place in a large bowl with the octopus. In a small bowl, combine the chile, garlic, lemon zest, and olive oil; season with salt and pepper to taste. Add half the chile mixture to the shrimp and octopus; toss to coat in the mixture. Cover and refrigerate for 1 hour. Reserve, then refrigerate, the remaining chile mixture.

2 Meanwhile, make the dough. Place the bulgur in a heatproof bowl; cover with boiling water; let stand, covered, for 30 minutes. Rinse under cold water; drain. In a small bowl, combine 1/2 cup of warm water, sugar, and yeast, cover; leave in a warm place for 10 minutes or until frothy. In a medium bowl, combine the bulgur, all-purpose flour, and whole wheat flour. Add the yeast mixture; mix to a soft dough. Knead the dough on a floured surface for 5 minutes or until smooth and elastic. Place the dough in an oiled medium bowl. Cover; let stand in a warm place for 45 minutes or until doubled in size.

3 Preheat oven to 425°F (220°C). Lightly oil two baking sheets.

4 Divide the dough into four pieces. Roll each piece into a disc 6in (15cm) in diameter; place each one on a baking sheet. Bake these pizza bases for 8 minutes or until partially cooked. Top with the seafood mixture and tomatoes. Bake the pizzas for 10 additional minutes or until the bases are crisp and the seafood is just cooked. Drizzle with the reserved chile mixture.

5 In a small bowl, combine the arugula and lemon juice; toss gently to coat. Season with salt and pepper to taste.

6 Top pizzas with the arugula mixture; serve with lemon wedges.

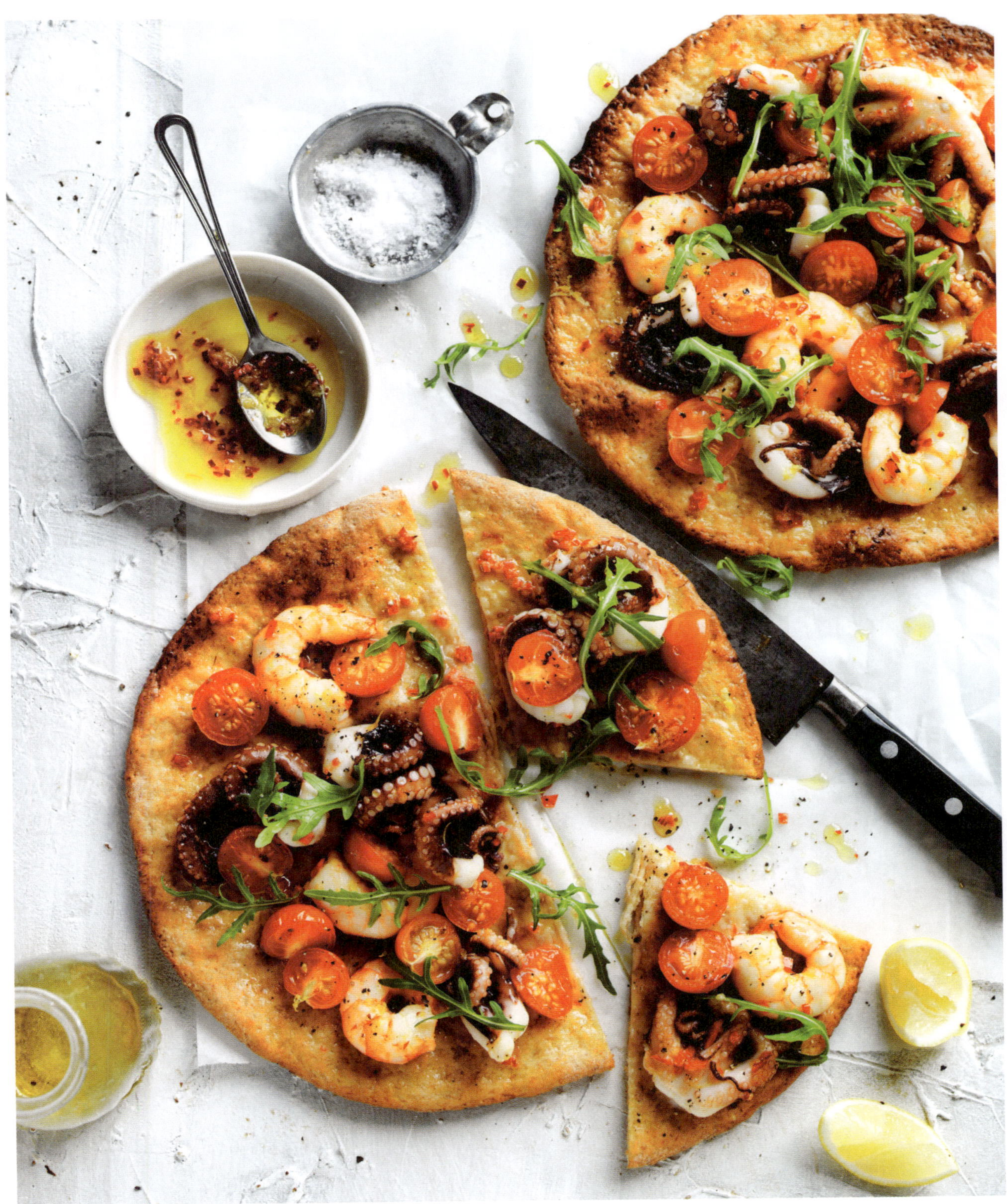

Lamb kefta, white bean, and beet tzatziki

PREP + COOK TIME **40 MINUTES** | SERVES **4**

Beets are notable for their distinct red color and earthy, sweet flavor. They're a good source of iron and folate, and also contain nitrates, betaine, magnesium, and other antioxidants. More recent health claims suggest beets can help lower blood pressure, boost exercise performance, and prevent dementia.

1 x 15oz (425g) can butter beans or Great Northern beans, drained, rinsed
1 tbsp lemon juice
2 tbsp fresh oregano leaves
2 tbsp olive oil, divided
salt and freshly ground black pepper
1/2 cup fresh breadcrumbs
2 tbsp milk
1 1/2lb (600g) ground lamb
1 tsp ground allspice
1/3 cup fresh oregano, extra, roughly chopped
1/2 cup feta cheese, crumbled
1 small head Romaine lettuce, leaves separated
lemon slices, for serving

beet tzatziki

1 medium beet, peeled, coarsely grated (about 3/4 cup)
1 cup Greek yogurt
2 tbsp chopped fresh mint leaves
1 garlic clove, crushed
1 tbsp finely grated lemon zest

TIPS

- If you don't have metal skewers, thread kefta onto bamboo skewers that have been soaked in water for 10 minutes to prevent them from burning during cooking.
- Cooked or uncooked kefta can be frozen for up to 3 months; thaw in the fridge.

1. To make the beet tzatziki, combine the ingredients in a medium bowl; season with salt and pepper to taste.
2. Combine the butter beans, lemon juice, oregano leaves, and 1 tbsp of the olive oil in a medium bowl; season with salt and pepper to taste.
3. Place the breadcrumbs and milk in a medium bowl; let stand for 3 minutes or until the milk has been absorbed. Add the lamb, allspice, and extra oregano; season with salt and pepper. Using your hands, work the mixture until well combined. Add the feta cheese; mix until combined. Roll heaped tablespoon measures of the lamb mixture—which is called kefta—into ball shapes. Thread onto 8 skewers.
4. Heat the remaining oil in a large nonstick sauté pan over medium-high heat; cook the kefta, turning occasionally, for 10 minutes or until browned and cooked through. If serving with lemon slices, add them to the pan with the kefta until pan fried.
5. Serve the kefta on the lettuce with the bean mixture, the beet tzatziki, and pan-fried lemon slices, if using.

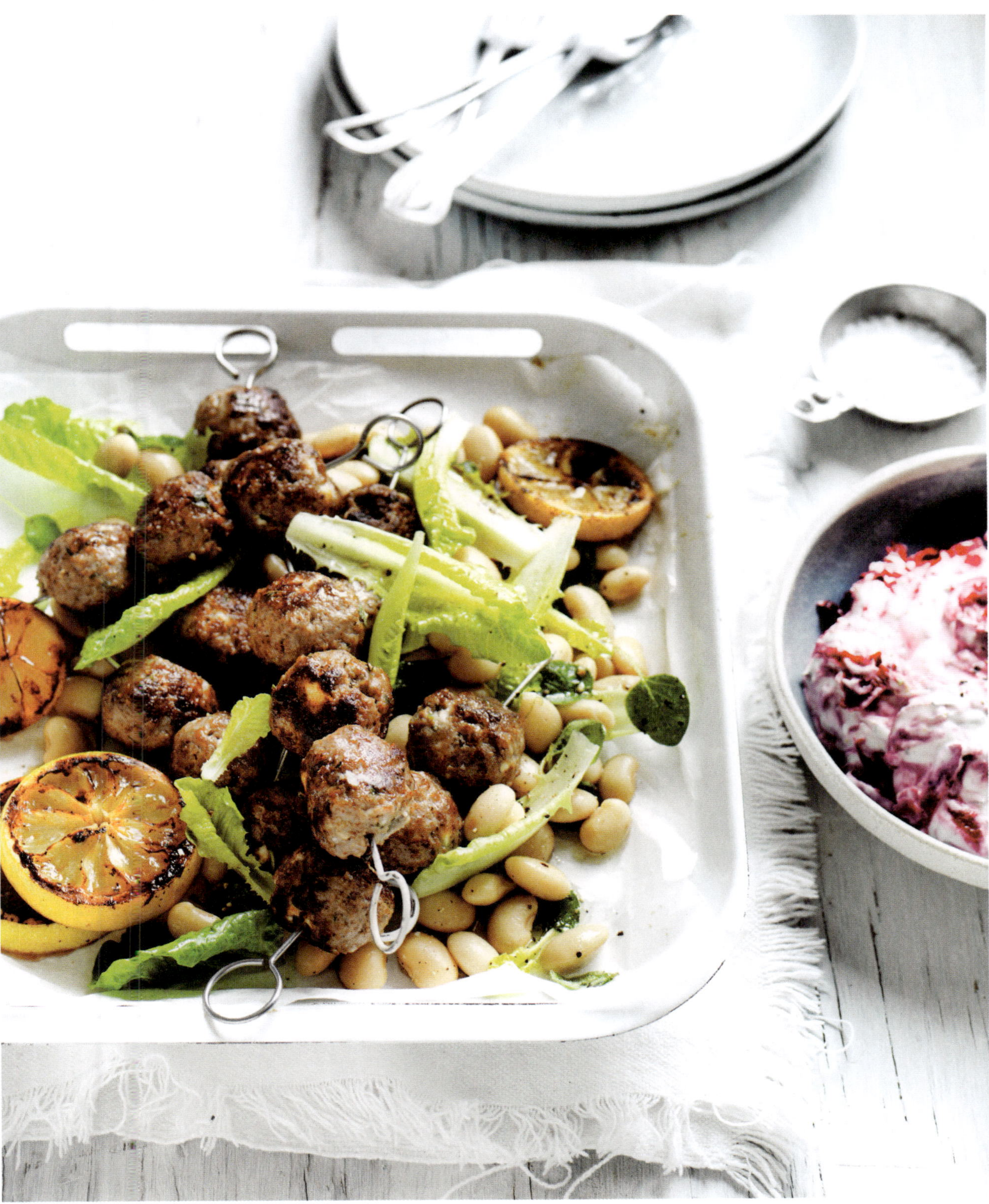

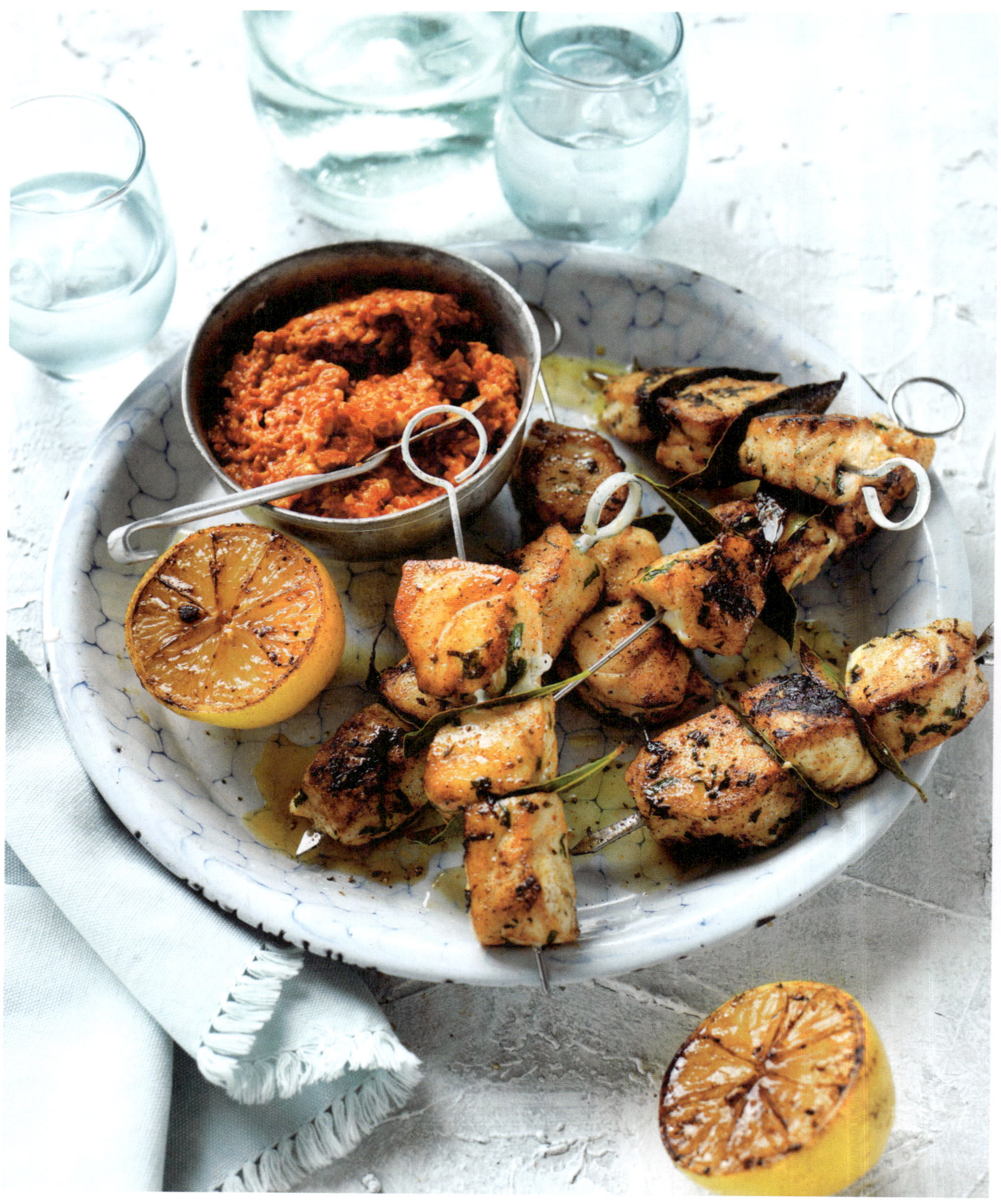

Spanish fish skewers with smoky romesco sauce

PESCATARIAN | PREP + COOK TIME **1 HOUR 45 MINUTES + COOLING AND REFRIGERATION** | SERVES **4**

Romesco is a traditional northern Spanish sauce, much like pesto in texture, made from a mixture of nuts and fire-roasted peppers. It often accompanies fish and seafood. Romesco also goes well with barbecued meats or chargrilled vegetables such as eggplant and zucchini.

2 red bell peppers, seeded and quartered
3 garlic cloves, unpeeled
1½ lb (350g) skinless boneless firm white fish fillets (bluefish, pompano, or Mediterranean sea bass), cut into 1in (2.5cm) pieces
2 tsp smoked paprika, divided
⅓ cup olive oil, divided
2 tsp finely grated lemon zest
2 tbsp fresh Italian parsley leaves, finely chopped
salt and freshly ground black pepper
24 fresh bay leaves
¼ cup blanched almonds
2 tbsp lemon juice
2 medium lemons, halved

1. Preheat the broiler and move the oven rack to a high position. Place the bell peppers, skin-side up, and the garlic on a baking sheet. Broil for 15 minutes or until the skins are blackened. Transfer to a medium bowl. Cover with plastic wrap and let the peppers steam for 20 minutes; let cool.
2. Combine the fish with 1 tsp of the smoked paprika, 3 tbsp of the olive oil, the lemon zest, and parsley in a medium bowl; season with salt and pepper. Thread the fish pieces onto 12 skewers with a bay leaf between each piece. Place the skewers on a baking sheet; cover, refrigerate.
3. Meanwhile, remove and discard skins from the red peppers and garlic cloves. In the bowl of a food processor, add the roasted red peppers, garlic, almonds, lemon juice, remaining paprika, and remaining olive oil; pulse until almost smooth. Transfer this romesco to a small bowl; season with salt and pepper to taste.
4. Cook the fish skewers in a large heavy-bottomed skillet or cast iron grill pan over medium-high heat for 4 minutes or until browned all over and cooked through. Add lemon halves to pan; cook for 1 minute or until browned.
5. Serve the fish skewers with the romesco sauce and cooked lemon halves.

TIPS

- You will need 12 bamboo or metal skewers for this recipe. Soak the bamboo skewers for 10 minutes in water before using to prevent them from burning during cooking; oil metal skewers to prevent sticking.
- Romesco can be made a day ahead; keep covered in the fridge.

Pan con tomate

VEGETARIAN | PREP + COOK TIME **15 MINUTES** | SERVES **2**

Pan con tomate—or bread with tomato—is a staple breakfast in Spain and is a humble dish full of robust flavors. The key is to have summer-ripe tomatoes, good-quality bread, and delicious olive oil. You could serve this as an appetizer at a party, or pair with a hearty salad for a light summer dinner. Serve topped with a fried or soft-boiled egg for a delicious twist.

10oz (285g) cherry tomatoes (see tip)
1/4 cup olive oil
salt and freshly ground black pepper
4 large slices sourdough bread
1 garlic clove, halved
2 1/2 oz (70g) goat cheese, crumbled
2 tbsp fresh oregano leaves

1. Preheat oven to 400°F (200°C). Line a baking sheet with parchment paper.
2. Place the tomatoes on the baking sheet, drizzle with 2 tbsp of olive oil; season with salt and pepper. Roast for 10 minutes or until the skins burst and the tomatoes have softened.
3. Drizzle the bread with the remaining olive oil. Grill the bread on a preheated ridged grill pan for 1 minute each side or until lightly charred. Rub the grilled bread slices with the cut side of the garlic.
4. Top the toasted bread with the roasted tomatoes, pressing down to break the tomatoes open and release their juice. Top with the goat cheese and oregano.

TIP

Cherry tomatoes with the stems still attached are called "on the vine". The stem isn't edible, but looks lovely when presenting this dish to guests.

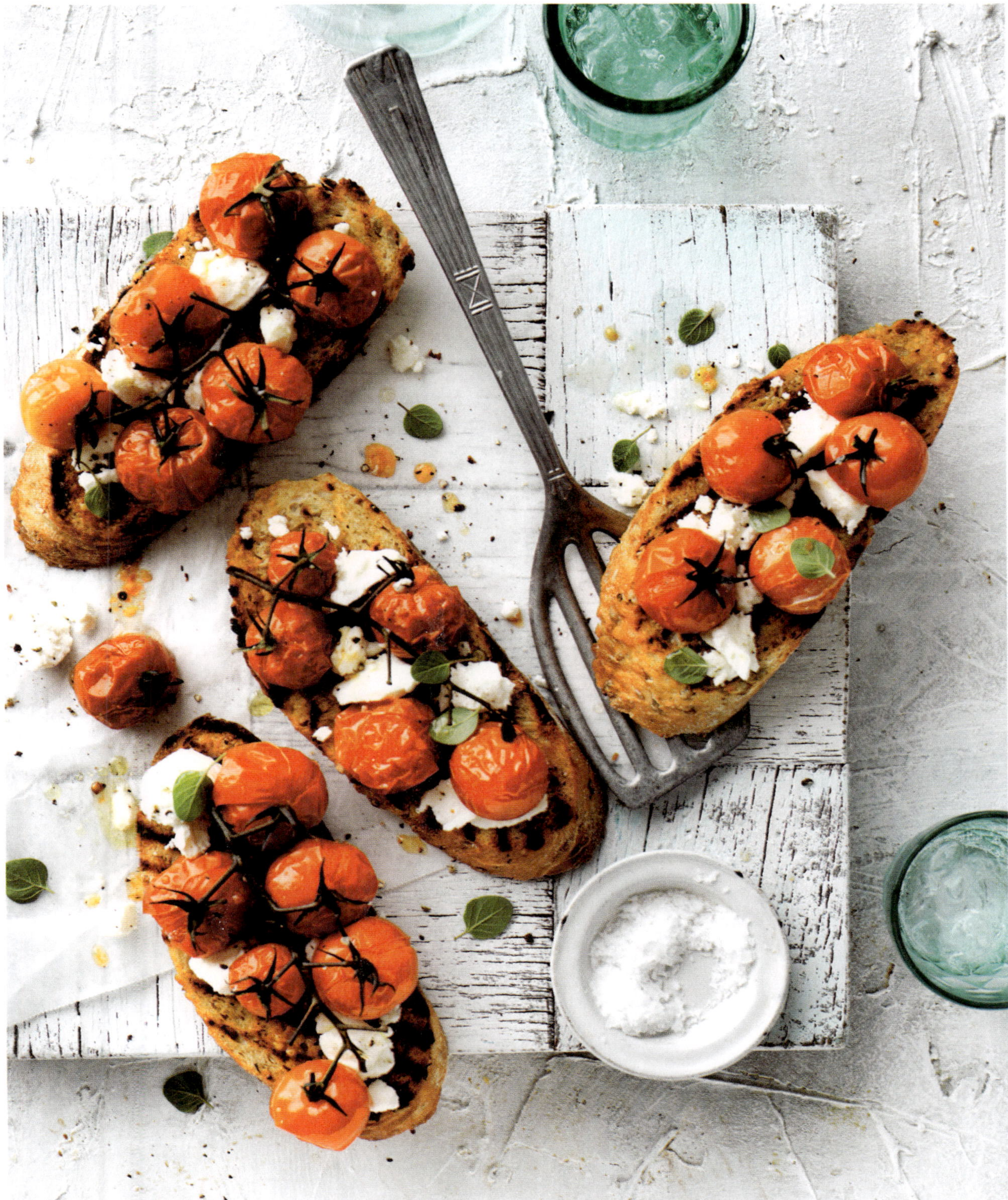

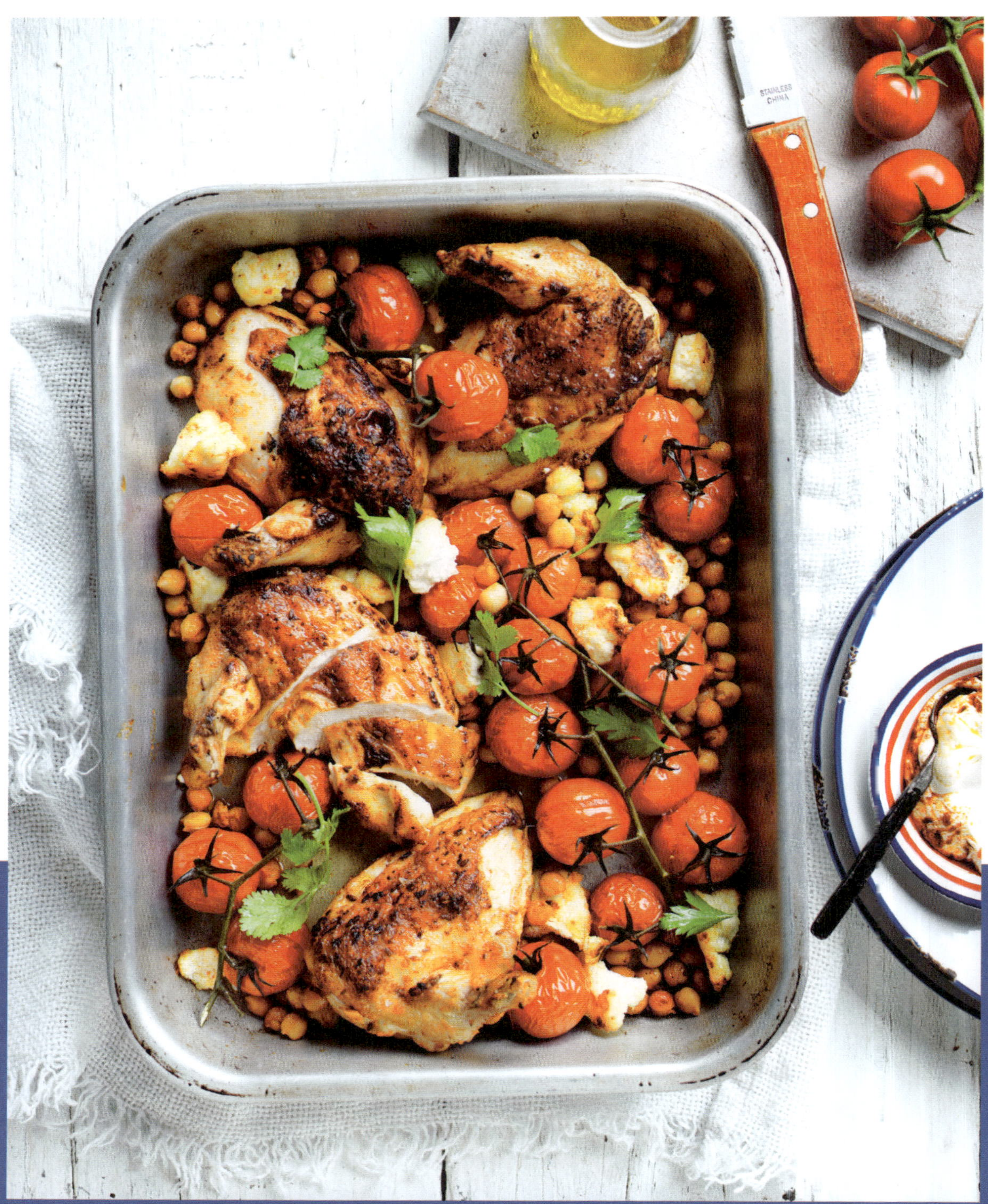
STAINLESS
CHINA

FAMILY TABLE

These delicious dishes are designed to be shared around a communal table with family and friends—a philosophy that lies at the heart of Mediterranean eating.

Savory cumin beans

VEGAN | PREP + COOK TIME **1 HOUR 20 MINUTES + OVERNIGHT SOAKING** | SERVES **6**

Beans are a great vegan option packed with protein and fiber. Dried beans give a better flavor and texture than canned ones, though canned beans will work fine in this recipe. Take leftover baked beans to work for a delicious lunch that has none of the added sugar or salt of the more traditional versions.

8oz (225g) dried cannellini or Great Northern beans
2 tbsp olive oil
2 medium onions, finely chopped (about 1½ cups)
8 garlic cloves, thinly sliced
1 tsp ground cumin
2 fresh long red chiles, thinly sliced
¼ cup tomato paste
3 medium tomatoes, roughly chopped
2 cups vegetable stock
2 tbsp fresh oregano, roughly chopped
salt and freshly ground black pepper
grilled sourdough bread, for serving
fresh oregano leaves, for serving

1. Place the beans in a large bowl, cover with cold water; let soak overnight. Drain. Rinse under cold water; drain.
2. Place the beans in a medium saucepan, cover with water; bring to a boil over high heat. Boil for 30 minutes or until the beans are almost tender. Drain.
3. Heat the olive oil in a large heavy-bottomed saucepan over medium heat. Add the onion, garlic, cumin, and chile; cook, stirring occasionally, for 7 minutes or until the onion is golden. Add the tomato paste, tomatoes, and stock; bring to a boil. Reduce heat to medium; cook, covered, for 10 minutes or until the sauce thickens slightly.
4. Add the beans to the pan; cook, covered, for 10 minutes, stirring occasionally. Remove lid; cook for 10 minutes or until the beans are tender. Stir in the chopped oregano; season with salt and pepper to taste.
5. Serve cumin baked beans with grilled bread and fresh oregano, if desired.

TIP

You will need to start this recipe the day before if you're soaking dried beans. Or save time by using 2 x 15 oz (425g) cans cannellini or Great Northern beans, drained and rinsed.

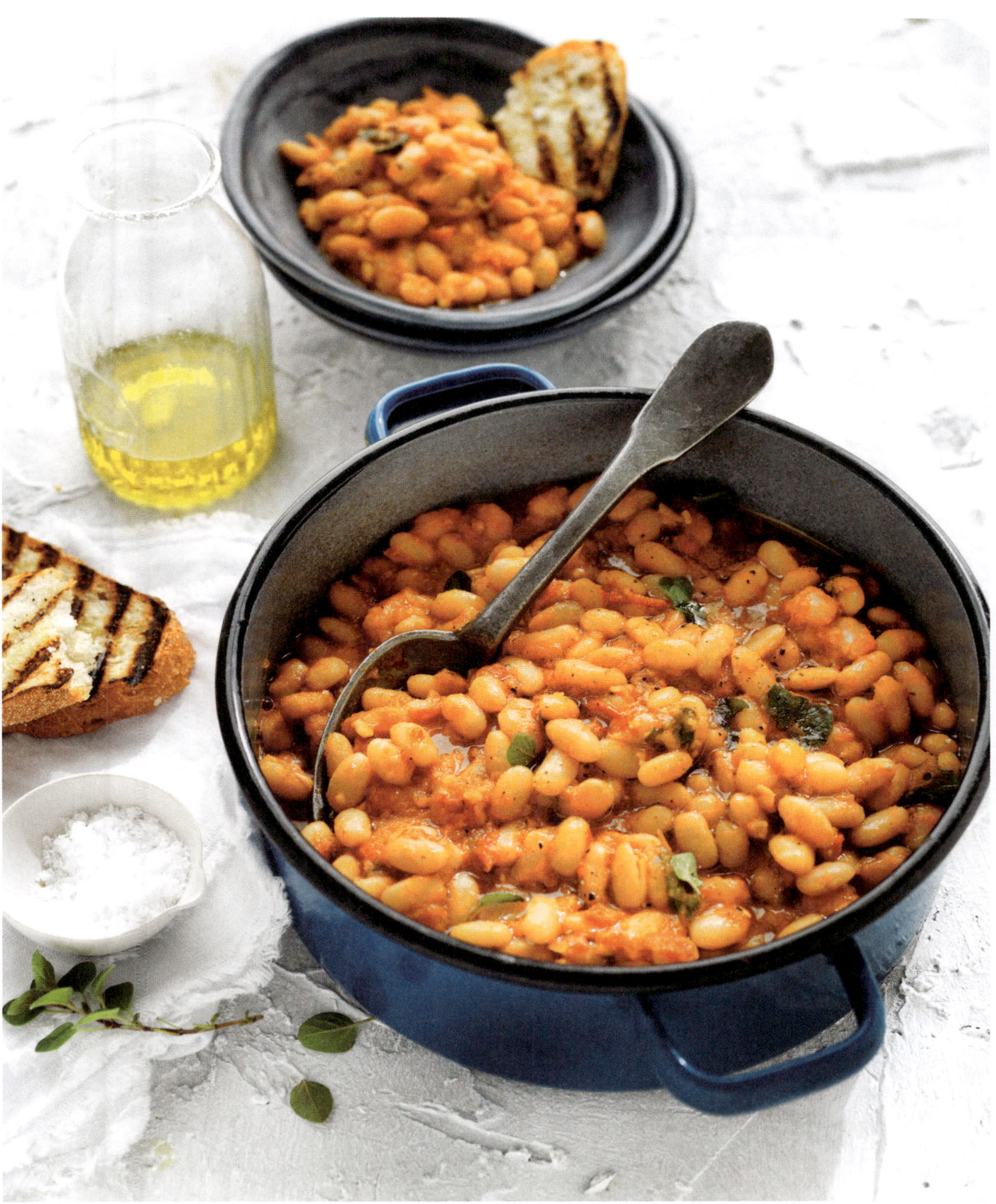

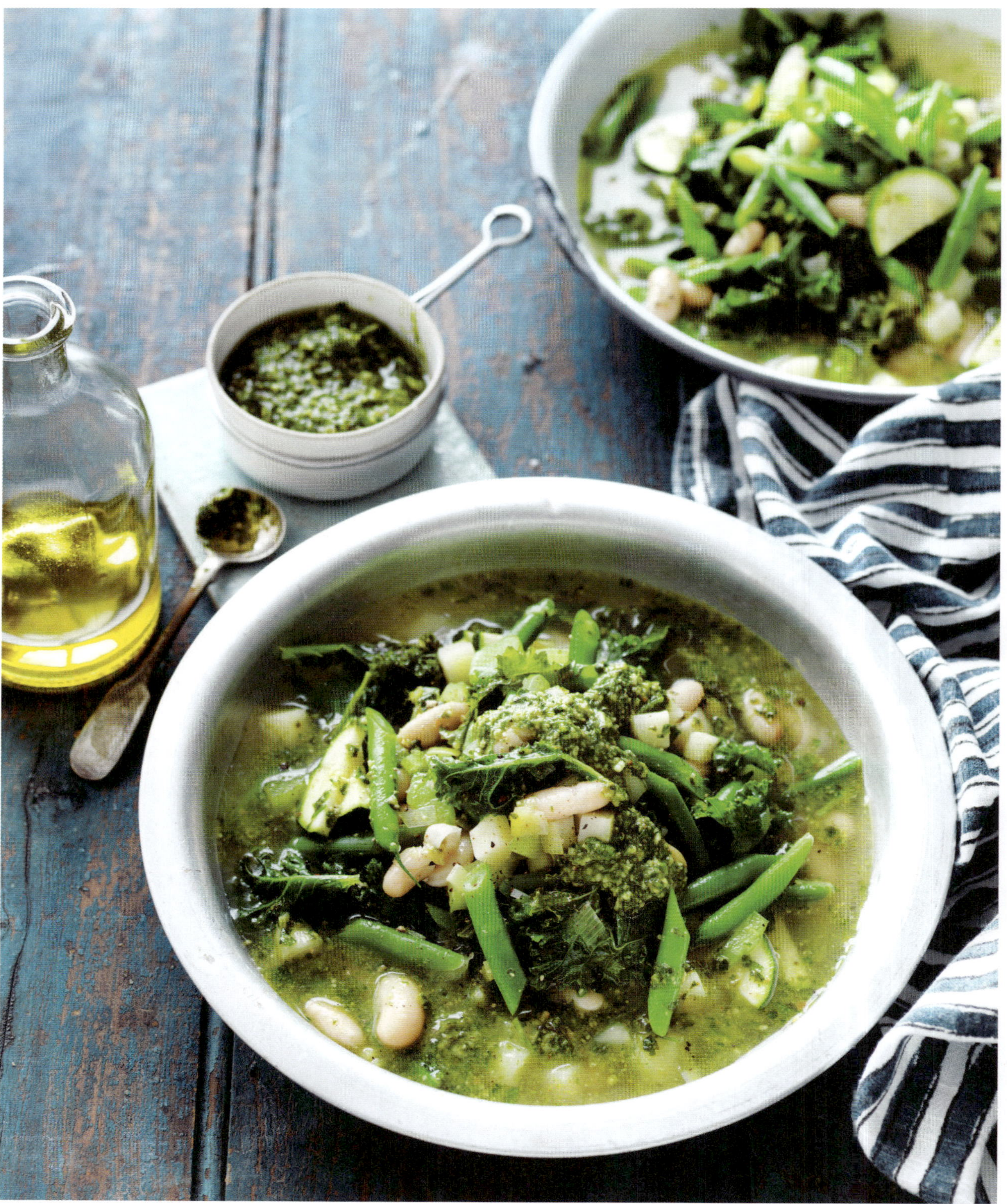

Green minestrone with pesto

VEGETARIAN | PREP + COOK TIME **35 MINUTES** | SERVES **4**

There is no set recipe for minestrone, which is traditionally made with whatever vegetables are in season at the time of cooking. The soup frequently contains cranberry beans, but this version instead uses cannellini beans and substitutes pesto and bright green vegetables for the traditional tomatoes.

2 tbsp olive oil

1 tsp fresh sage leaves, finely chopped

2 garlic cloves, finely chopped

1 medium leek, finely chopped

1 medium parsnip, peeled, cut into 1/2 in (1cm) cubes

2 celery stalks, trimmed, thinly sliced

3 cups curly kale, stems discarded, torn into pieces

6 cups vegetable stock

1/4 lb (150g) green beans, trimmed, cut diagonally into 1in (2.5cm) pieces

1 large zucchini, halved lengthways, thinly sliced

1 x 15oz (425g) can cannellini or Great Northern beans, drained, rinsed

salt and freshly ground black pepper

pesto

2 cups fresh basil leaves

1/3 cup finely grated Parmesan cheese

1/4 cup pine nuts, toasted

1/2 garlic clove, peeled

1/2 cup olive oil

1. Heat the olive oil in a large saucepan over medium heat. Cook the sage, garlic, and leek, stirring, for 3 minutes or until the leek is soft. Add the parsnip, celery, and kale; cook, stirring, for 2 minutes or until the kale is bright green. Add the stock, bring to a boil; reduce heat to low. Simmer for 15 minutes or until the parsnip is almost tender.
2. Add the green beans, zucchini, and cannellini beans; cook for 5 minutes or until the green beans are tender. Season with salt and pepper to taste.
3. Meanwhile, make the pesto. Place all of the ingredients into the bowl of a food processor. Pulse until smooth. Transfer to a small bowl; season with salt and pepper to taste.
4. Ladle the soup into bowls. Serve topped with the pesto.

TIPS

- The soup can be made a day ahead; keep covered in the fridge.
- The pesto can be made 3 days ahead; keep tightly covered, in a small airtight container, in the fridge. If it dries out, add a little more olive oil.

Spaghettini niçoise

PESCATARIAN | PREP + COOK TIME **30 MINUTES** | SERVES **4**

This riff on salad niçoise, a classic French favorite, is equally enjoyable served warm or room temperature. Easy to prepare in advance, it's a great addition to your repertoire of workday lunches and makes excellent picnic fare. Omit the chile if you like.

8oz (225g) spaghettini or thin spaghetti

4 eggs

½lb (225g) fresh tuna steak, grilled or pan seared, and flaked into chunks (see tip)

⅓ cup pitted Kalamata olives, roughly chopped

10oz (285g) cherry tomatoes, halved

⅓ cup pine nuts, toasted

1 cup arugula

salt and freshly ground black pepper

½ tsp dried chile flakes

lemon mustard dressing

2 tbsp olive oil

1 tbsp finely grated lemon zest

¼ cup lemon juice

1 garlic clove, crushed

1 tbsp Dijon mustard

1 tbsp nonpareil capers

1. Make the lemon mustard dressing. Place all of the ingredients in a screw-top jar; shake well. Season with salt and pepper to taste.
2. Cook the pasta in a large pot of boiling salted water until almost tender; drain. Return to pot.
3. Meanwhile, place the eggs in a small saucepan, cover with cold water; bring to a boil. Cook for 2 minutes or until soft-boiled; drain. Rinse under cold water; drain. When cool enough to handle, peel the eggs.
4. Add the tuna, olives, tomatoes, pine nuts, arugula, and dressing to the pasta in the pot; toss gently. Season with salt and pepper to taste.
5. Serve the pasta topped with halved soft-boiled eggs and chile flakes.

TIP

Grilled tuna makes this a hearty dish, but if it's not available, use 2 x 5oz (140g) cans of white albacore tuna—or a high-quality tuna—packed in olive oil.

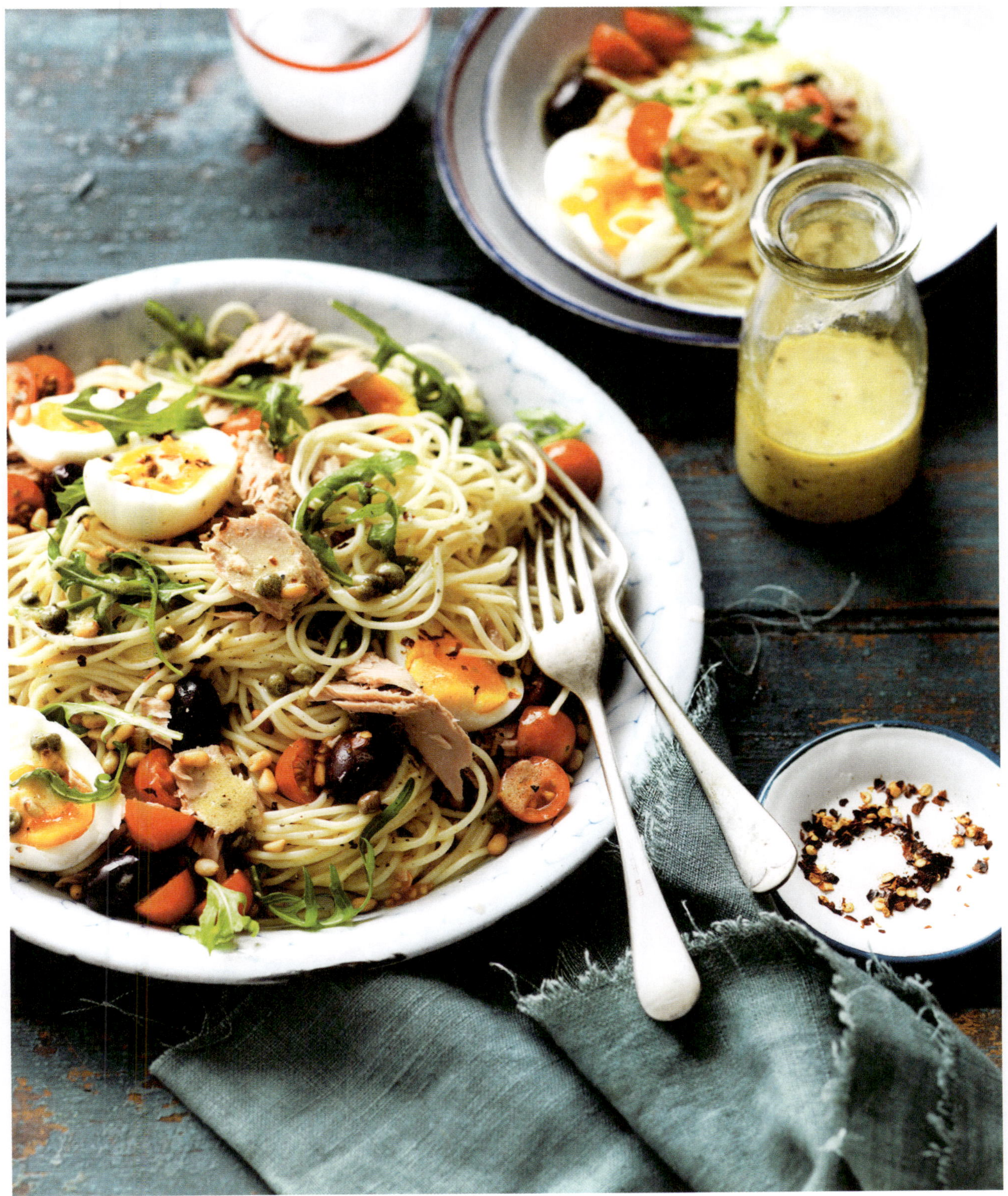

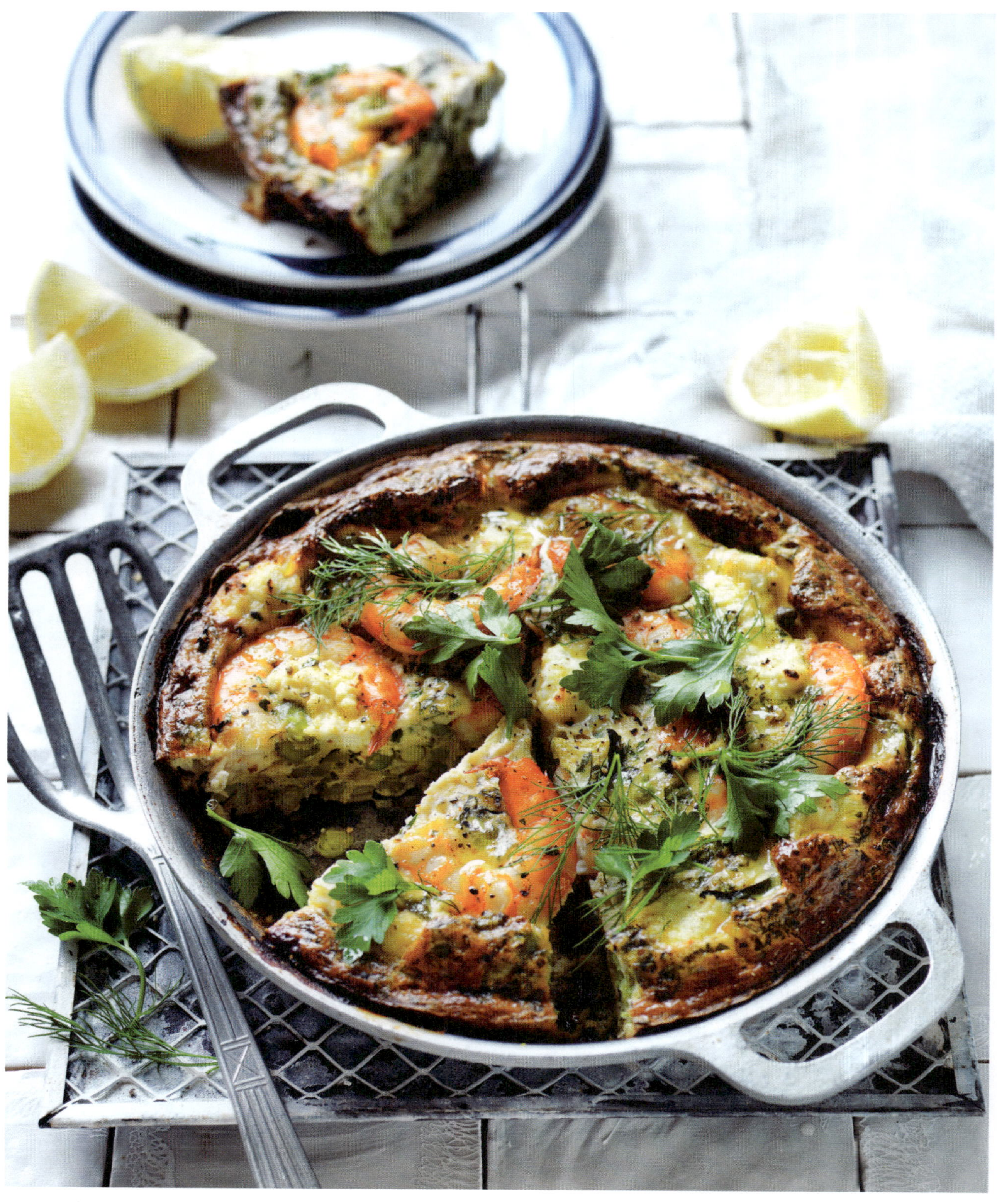

Shrimp, pea, and fava bean frittata

PESCATARIAN | PREP + COOK TIME **1 HOUR** | SERVES **4**

Derived from the Italian word *friggere,* which roughly translates as "fried," a frittata is an amazingly versatile dish—the perfect vehicle for using up leftovers, while relatively simple to cook. It also makes the best packed lunch for work or school, as it can be eaten heated or cool. Serve with a simple green salad for a complete meal.

- 1/2 cup fresh Italian parsley leaves, divided
- 1/3 cup fresh dill, divided
- 6 eggs
- 1/2 cup buttermilk
- 2 tbsp dry breadcrumbs
- salt and freshly ground black pepper
- 1/2 lb (225g) fresh or frozen fava beans
- 2 tbsp extra virgin olive oil
- 1 large zucchini, halved lengthwise, thinly sliced
- 3 spring onions, thinly sliced
- 2 garlic cloves, crushed
- 2 cups frozen peas, thawed
- 1lb (500g) cooked medium shrimp, peeled, deveined
- 1/3 cup ricotta cheese
- lemon halves, for serving

1. Coarsely chop half the herbs; reserve the remaining herbs. Whisk the chopped herbs, eggs, buttermilk, and breadcrumbs in a large bowl; season with salt and pepper.
2. Cook the fava beans in a large saucepan of boiling water for 2 minutes or until just tender; drain. Place under cold running water to stop the cooking, drain well. Remove gray skins.
3. Preheat oven to 350°F (180°C).
4. Heat the olive oil in an 8in (21cm) ovenproof skillet over medium heat; cook the zucchini and spring onion, stirring, for 5 minutes or until soft. Add the garlic, peas, and fava beans; cook, stirring, for 1 minute or until fragrant. Add the egg mixture, gently shake pan to distribute mixture; reduce heat to low-medium. Cook, without stirring, for 5 minutes or until the edge is set. Top with the shrimp and crumbled ricotta cheese.
5. Bake the frittata for 20 minutes or until the center is just firm.
6. Serve the frittata with the remaining herbs and the lemon halves.

TIP

You can also use dried fava beans. Simply cook them according to the package instructions.

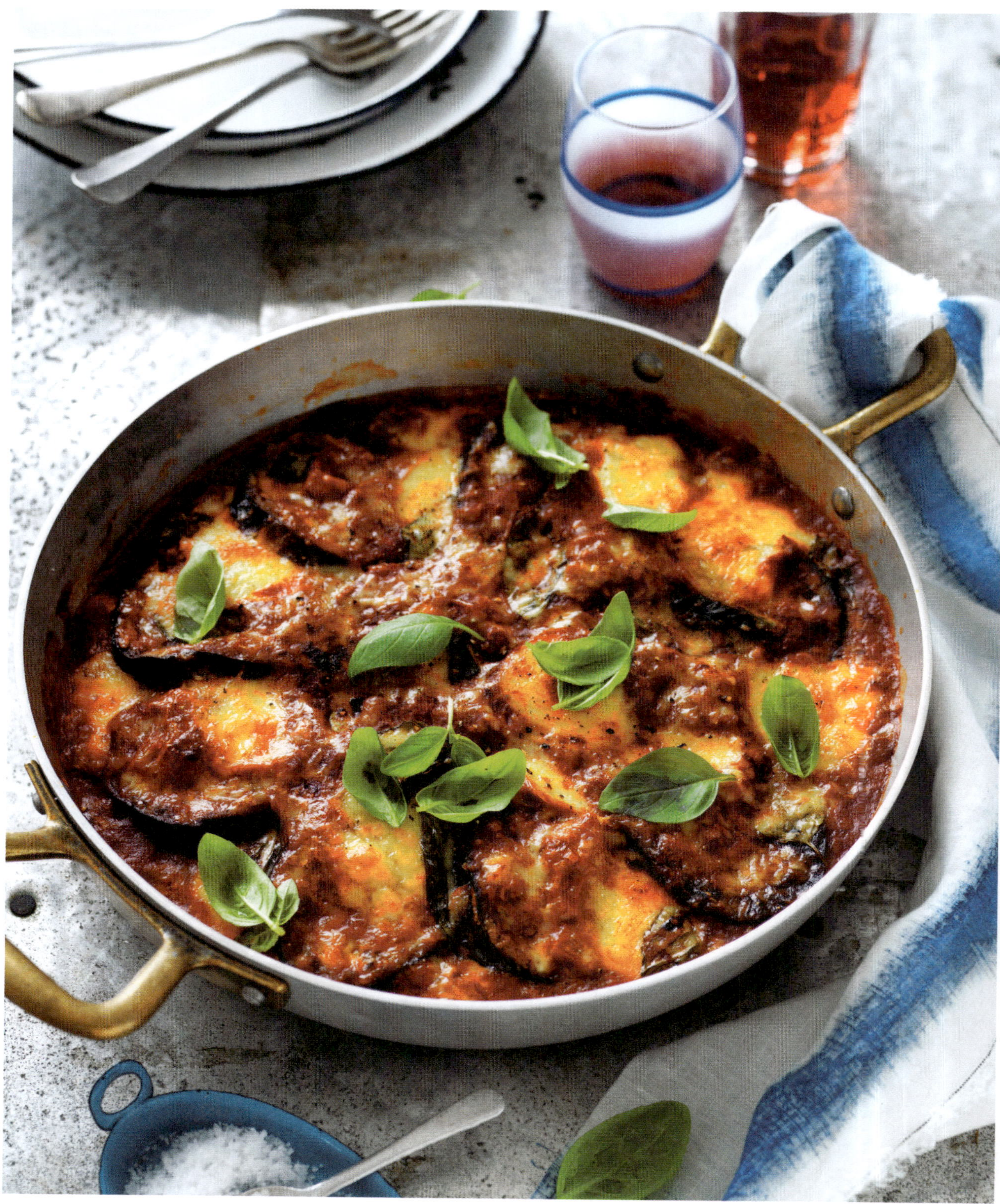

Eggplant parmigiana

VEGETARIAN | PREP + COOK TIME **1 HOUR 15 MINUTES** | SERVES **4**

Serve this satisfying Italian layered dish with a salad and crusty bread, or stir through cooked short pasta. Look for bocconcini mozzarella—baby mozzarella cheese balls, also called mozzarella "pearls" or "snacking cheese"—packed in liquid in the refrigerated cheese case.

- 2/3 cup olive oil
- 1 medium onion, finely chopped
- 2 garlic cloves, crushed
- 1 x 14.5oz (400g) can chopped tomatoes
- 1/4 tsp dried chile flakes
- salt and freshly ground black pepper
- 1 large eggplant, thickly sliced
- 1/4 cup all-purpose flour
- 1/3 cup fresh basil leaves
- 8oz (225g) bocconcini mozzarella, thinly sliced (see tip)
- 2/3 cup finely grated parmesan cheese
- 1/2 tsp sweet paprika
- small basil leaves, extra, to garnish

1. Preheat oven to 350°F (180°C).
2. Heat 1 tbsp of oil in a large frying pan over medium heat; cook onion, stirring, until soft. Add the garlic; cook, stirring, until fragrant. Stir in the tomatoes and chile; season with salt and pepper to taste. Transfer mixture to a medium jug.
3. Toss the eggplant in flour to coat; shake off excess. Heat the remaining olive oil in the same cleaned pan; cook the eggplant in batches, until browned on both sides. Drain on paper towel.
4. Spray a 9 x 9in (23 x 23cm) ovenproof baking dish with cooking spray. Layer 1/4 cup of the tomato mixture into the bottom of the dish. Layer half the eggplant slices on top of the tomato. Season with salt and pepper, then top with half of the remaining tomato mixture, the basil, and the mozzarella cheese. Repeat layering with the remaining eggplant, tomato mixture, and basil. Season with salt and pepper. Finish with the Parmesan cheese. Sprinkle with the sweet paprika.
5. Bake, covered, for 30 minutes. Uncover, bake for 15 more minutes or until browned and tender. Serve topped with the extra basil.

TIPS

You could also use the same amount of a full size mozzarella ball, cut into 1in (2.5cm) pieces, then sliced.

Roasted tomato soup with broccoli pesto

PREP + COOK TIME **1 HOUR + STANDING** | SERVES **4**

Tomatoes feature heavily in Mediterranean dishes, both in their raw state and cooked. While they are both nutritious and extremely tasty picked straight from the vine, cooking tomatoes increases their levels of lycopene, a phytochemical with significant antioxidant properties that's responsible for the bright red color of the vegetable.

2lb (1kg) vine-ripened tomatoes, quartered (see tip)
3 garlic cloves, unpeeled
3 sprigs fresh thyme
1 medium onion, chopped
salt and freshly ground black pepper
1/3 cup olive oil, divided
3 cups chicken stock
1 tbsp pine nuts, toasted
small fresh basil leaves, to garnish

broccoli pesto
2 cups broccoli florets, chopped
1 garlic clove, crushed
1 1/2 tbsp pine nuts, toasted
1 1/2 tbsp finely grated Parmesan cheese
1 1/2 tbsp fresh basil leaves, roughly chopped
1/4 cup olive oil

1. Preheat oven to 425°F (220°C). Line a baking sheet with parchment paper.
2. Place the tomatoes, garlic, thyme, and onion on the baking sheet; season with salt and pepper. Drizzle with 1/4 cup of the olive oil; toss to coat the tomatoes. Roast for 30 minutes or until the tomatoes are very soft and browned around the edges.
3. Meanwhile, make the broccoli pesto. Cook the broccoli in a small saucepan of boiling water for 2 minutes; drain. Run cold water over it to stop cooking; drain well. In the bowl of a food processor add the broccoli, garlic, pine nuts, Parmesan cheese, and basil. Pulse until finely chopped. With the processor running, gradually pour in the olive oil; process until combined. Season with salt and pepper to taste. Set aside.
4. Transfer the roasted tomatoes and onion to a medium saucepan. Remove the thyme stalks. Squeeze the garlic out of skins; add to the tomato mixture. Add the stock to the pan and bring to a boil. Cool for 10 minutes. Using a blender or food processor, pulse the soup until smooth; return the soup to the pan. Stir over a low heat until hot; season with salt and pepper to taste.
5. Ladle the soup into bowls; top with the broccoli pesto, pine nuts, and basil leaves. Drizzle with the remaining olive oil.

TIPS

- Any fresh tomatoes will work, but Roma tomatoes, used for sauce, are particularly delicious in a soup like this one.
- The soup and the broccoli pesto can be frozen, separately, for up to 3 months.

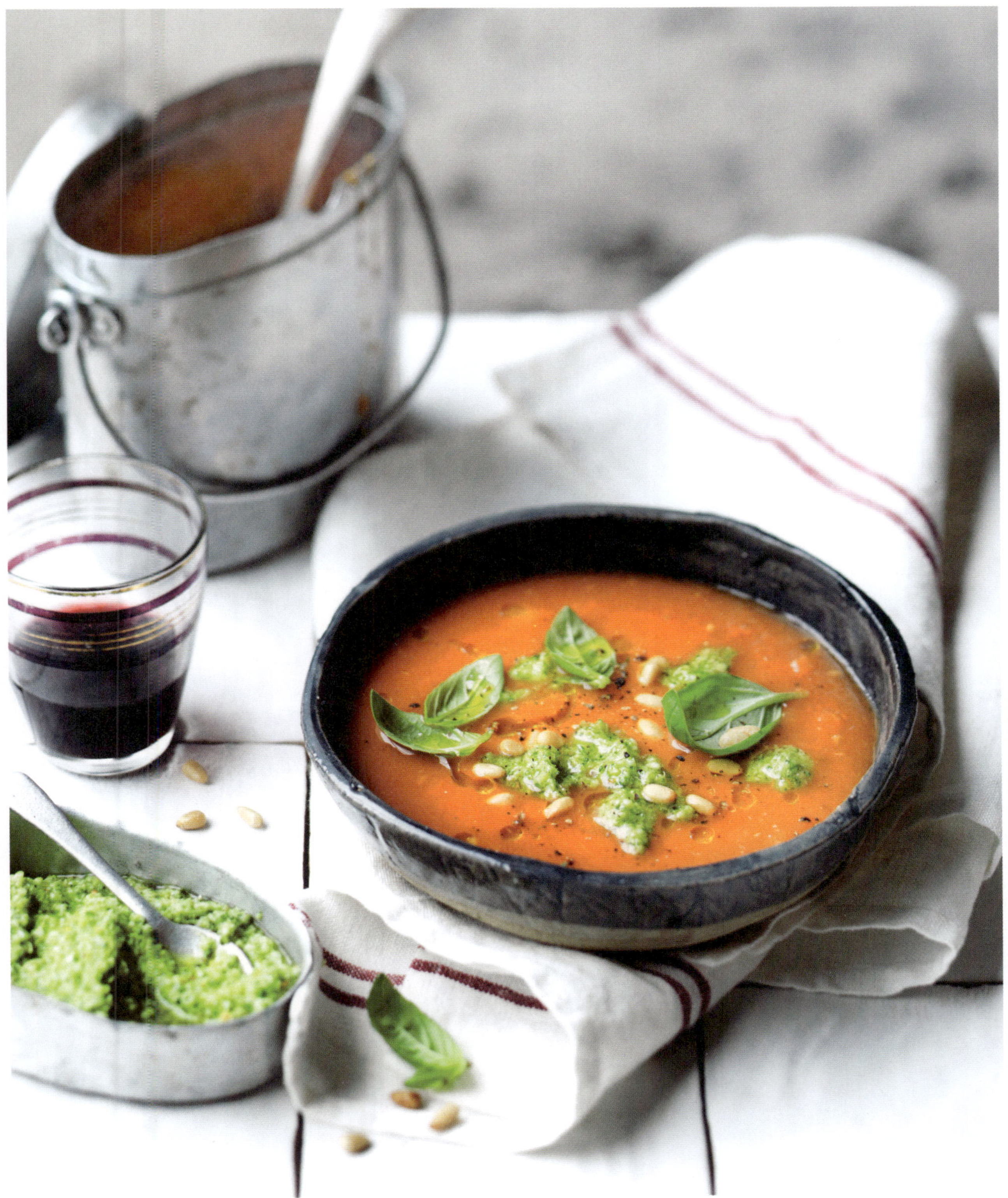

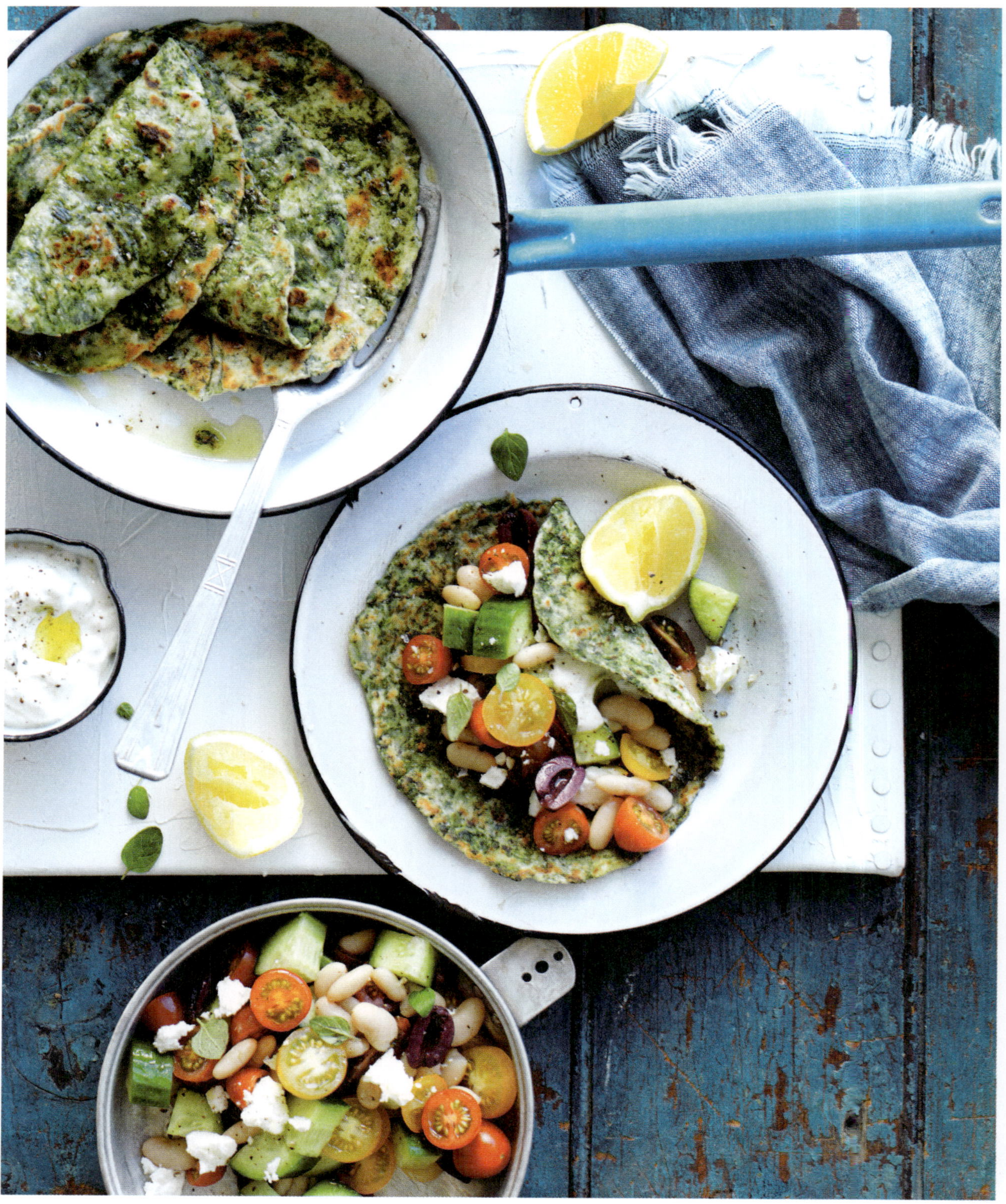

Spinach and yogurt flatbread with Greek bean salad

VEGETARIAN | PREP + COOK TIME **45 MINUTES + STANDING** | SERVES **4**

Most people in the Mediterranean region can't imagine a day going by without consuming bread in one form or another. Fresh bread is surely one of the world's greatest comforts, and this simple recipe gives you a hassle-free way of preparing your own. This flatbread is perfect to accompany a light lunch or dinner, or to enjoy as a light meal on its own.

9oz (250g) frozen spinach, thawed, chopped
1 cup all-purpose flour
2 tsp baking powder
1/2 tsp salt
1/2 cup Greek yogurt
1 garlic clove, crushed
salt and freshly ground black pepper
3 tbsp olive oil, divided
3/4 cup premade tzatziki (see tip)
lemon wedges, for serving

Greek bean salad

10oz (125g) cherry tomatoes, halved
1 medium cucumber, peeled, seeded, and chopped
1/2 cup canned cannellini or Great Northern beans, drained, rinsed
1/4 cup pitted black olives, halved
1/4 cup loosely packed fresh oregano leaves
4oz (100g) feta cheese, crumbled

1. Place the spinach in a clean cheesecloth. Squeeze over the sink to remove as much excess liquid as possible. Place the spinach, flour, baking powder, salt, yogurt, and garlic in a large bowl; season with salt and pepper. Use your hands to bring the ingredients together and form a rough dough. Cover; let dough stand for 1 hour.
2. Make the Greek bean salad. Place the ingredients in a large bowl; toss gently to combine. Season with salt and pepper to taste.
3. Divide the dough into eight balls. Roll out each ball of dough on a floured surface until 1/8in (2mm) thick.
4. Heat 1 tsp of the oil in a heavy-based skillet over medium heat. Add one of the flatbread dough balls and cook for 1 minute on each side or until golden. Remove from pan, cover to keep warm, or keep it warm in a preheated 275°F (130°C) oven. Repeat, adding 1 tsp of oil before each remaining ball of dough.
5. Top flatbreads evenly with tzatziki and salad; serve with lemon wedges.

TIPS

- If you can't find premade tzatziki, combine 1/2 cup plain Greek yogurt, half a cucumber (peeled, seeded, and chopped finely), and 2 tbsp lemon juice. Add garlic and fresh dill to taste if you wish.
- You can make the spinach dough a day ahead, cover, and refrigerate until needed. Bring to room temperature before rolling out.

Chicken, zucchini, and freekeh soup

PREP + COOK TIME **45 MINUTES** | SERVES **4**

Freekeh is made from roasted young green wheat. Nutritionally, freekeh stacks up impressively; it has a low GI and four times the fiber of brown rice, and is higher in protein than regular wheat. The name freekeh comes from the word *farik,* which refers to the way that freekeh is threshed, or "rubbed," to remove its tough and inedible outer bran layer.

½ cup cracked green-wheat freekeh (see tips)

1 tbsp olive oil

1 medium leek, white part only, halved, thinly sliced

4 garlic cloves, thinly sliced

5 cups water (see tips)

4 boneless chicken thighs

½ lb (150g) green beans, trimmed, cut into ¾in (2cm) lengths

salt and freshly ground black pepper

1 zucchini, halved lengthwise, thinly sliced

½ cup frozen peas

1 tsp finely grated lemon zest

2 tbsp lemon juice

2 tbsp chopped fresh Italian parsley leaves

1. Place the freekeh in a medium saucepan, cover with water; bring to a boil. Reduce heat to low; cook, partially covered, for 15 minutes or until almost tender. Drain. Set aside.
2. Meanwhile, heat the olive oil in a large saucepan over medium heat; cook the leek, stirring, for 4 minutes or until softened. Add the garlic; cook, stirring, for 2 minutes.
3. Add the water and chicken, bring to a boil; reduce heat to low. Cook, covered, for 12 minutes or until the chicken is cooked. Remove the chicken from the stock; shred the meat. Return the shredded chicken to the pan with the green beans and freekeh, season with salt and pepper to taste; cook for 5 minutes. Add the zucchini and peas; cook for 3 minutes or until tender. Stir in the lemon zest and juice.
4. Ladle the soup into bowls; top with parsley. Season with salt and pepper to taste.

TIPS

- Freekeh is a wheat product so it does contain gluten; it is available from health food stores and some supermarkets.
- For a more intense flavor, use homemade chicken stock instead of water.

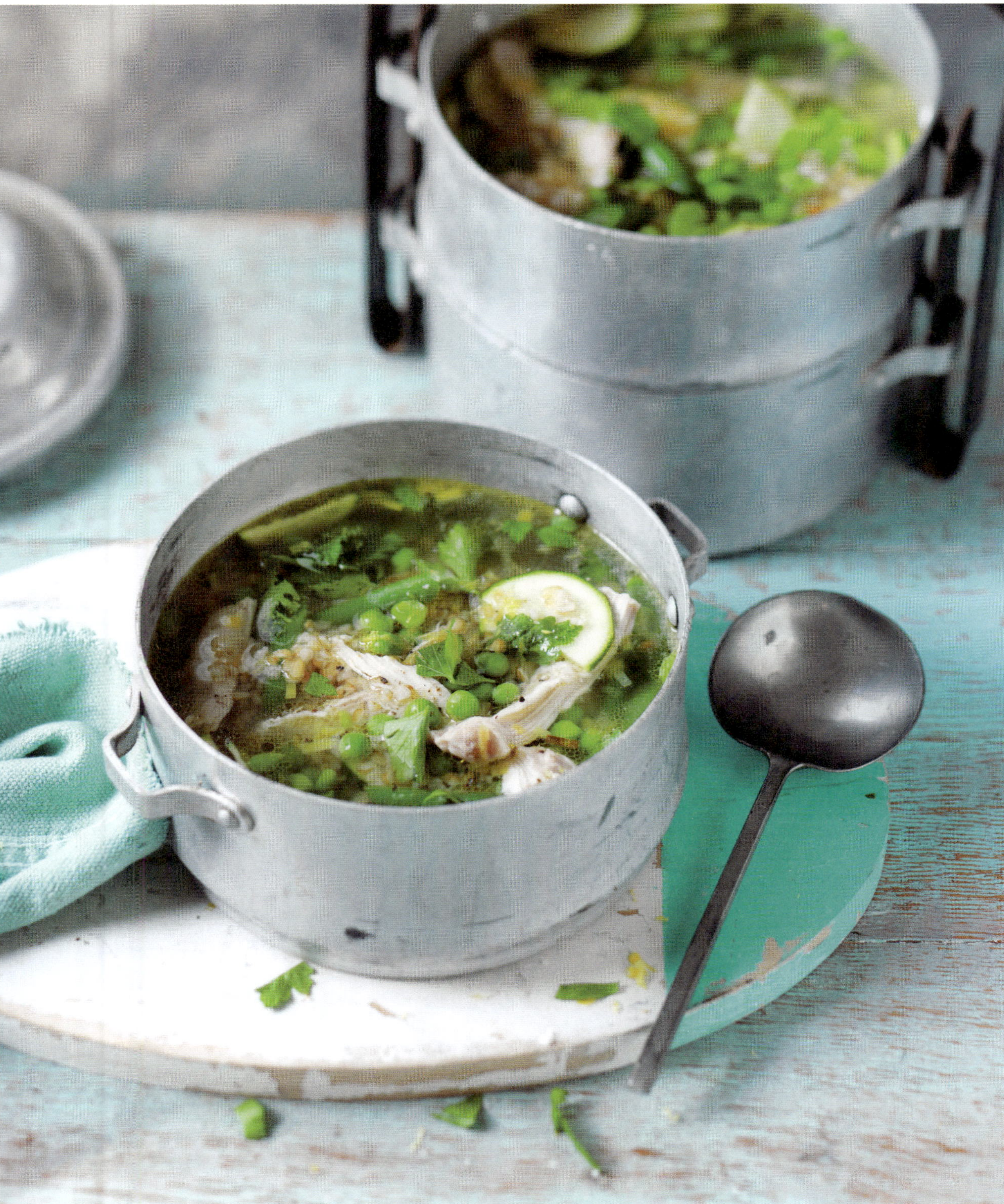

Mushrooms

Mushrooms are a great source of fiber, protein, vitamin C, B vitamins, calcium, minerals, and selenium. Studies have shown they can help to reduce blood pressure and cholesterol, enhance the immune system, and assist in fighting many types of cancer.

Mushroom with almond picada

VEGAN | PREP + COOK TIME **45 MINUTES** | SERVES **2**

Preheat the oven to 400°F (200°C). In a food processor, add 1 slice of day-old bread, 1 chopped garlic clove, 1/4 cup natural almonds, and 1/2 cup fresh Italian parsley and pulse until coarsely chopped. Scatter the mixture over 6 medium portobello mushroom caps and 10oz (250g) of grape tomatoes on a parchment paper-lined baking sheet. Drizzle with 1/4 cup olive oil. Cover with foil. Bake for 15 minutes. Remove foil; bake for 15 minutes more or until tender. Serve sprinkled with lemon zest and chopped fresh chile.

Mushroom crostini

VEGETARIAN | PREP TIME **20 MINUTES** | MAKES **4**

Peel 4 medium-sized portobello mushrooms, trim stalks level with the cap. Brush one side of 4 thick slices of sourdough bread with a little olive oil. Place slices, oiled-side down, on a hot grill or ridged grill pan; cook until lightly toasted. Stuff/fill each mushroom cap with 2 tbsp of pesto; place the mushrooms on bread on the grill or grill pan. Cover with parchment paper. Cook for 5 minutes or until the mushrooms are tender and the bread is golden. Top mushrooms with 1/2 cup of crumbled feta cheese; drizzle with a little olive oil. Serve with lemon wedges.

Mushroom and dill pilaf

VEGAN | PREP + COOK TIME **20 MINUTES** | SERVES **2**

Heat 2 tbsp of olive oil in a frying pan over high heat; cook 1/2 lb (250g) cremini or baby portobello mushrooms for 8 minutes or until browned and tender. Remove from the pan. To the pan, add 1 cup cooked brown basmati rice, 2 finely chopped spring onions, 1 tsp smoked paprika, and 2 tbsp each of pistachios and currants; cook, stirring, for 5 minutes or until heated through. Stir in 1/2 cup roughly chopped dill and the mushrooms.

Mushroom and radicchio salad

VEGETARIAN | PREP TIME **15 MINUTES** | SERVES **4**

Heat 2 tbsp of olive oil in a large frying pan over high heat; cook 3 cups mixed wild mushrooms (including oyster mushrooms, chanterelles, and morels) and 2 tsp of thyme leaves, stirring occasionally, for 5 minutes or until browned. Remove from the pan; cool. In a large bowl, whisk 1 1/2 tbsp each of balsamic vinegar and olive oil. Add half a head of torn radicchio leaves, the mushrooms, and 2 tbsp each of pumpkin seeds and shaved Parmesan cheese; toss gently to combine.

CLOCKWISE from top left

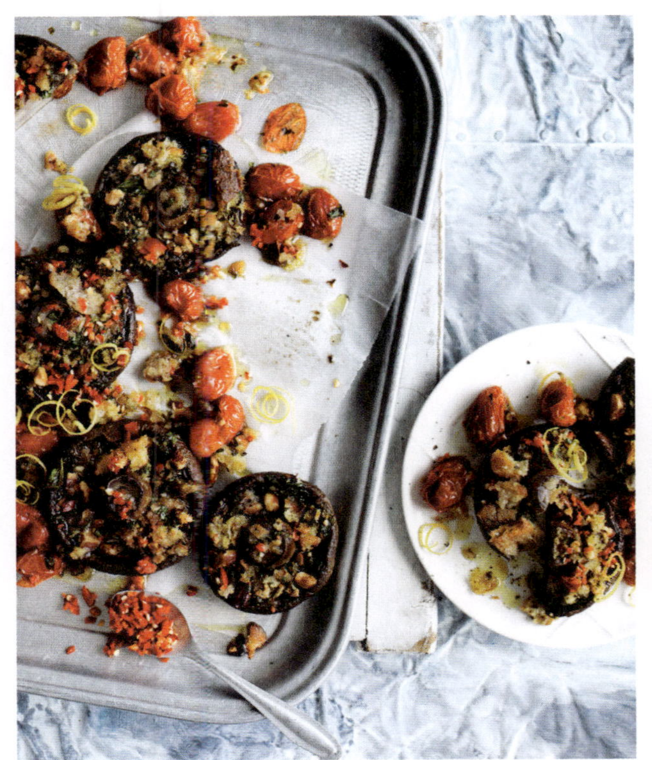

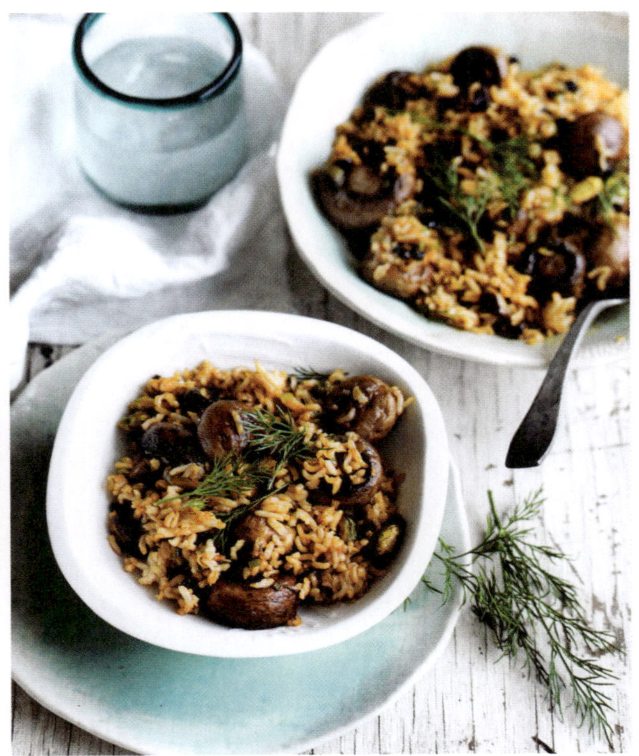

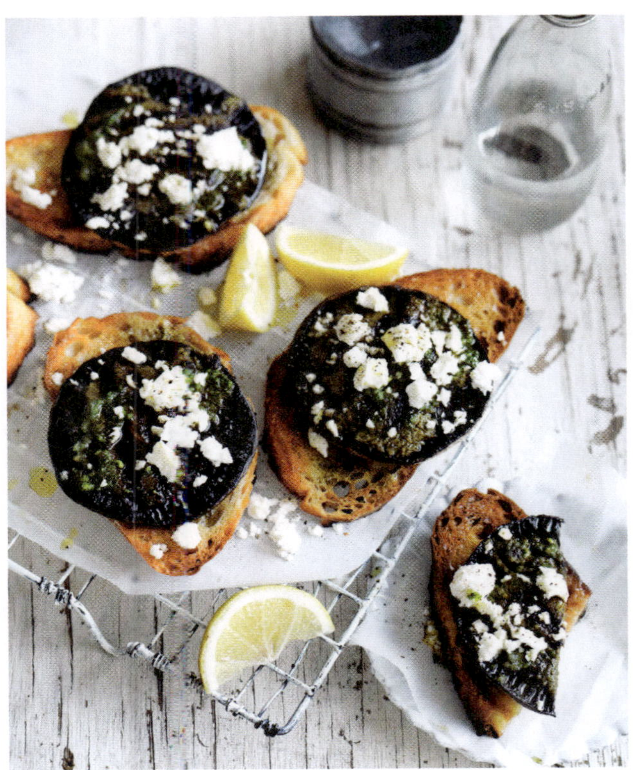

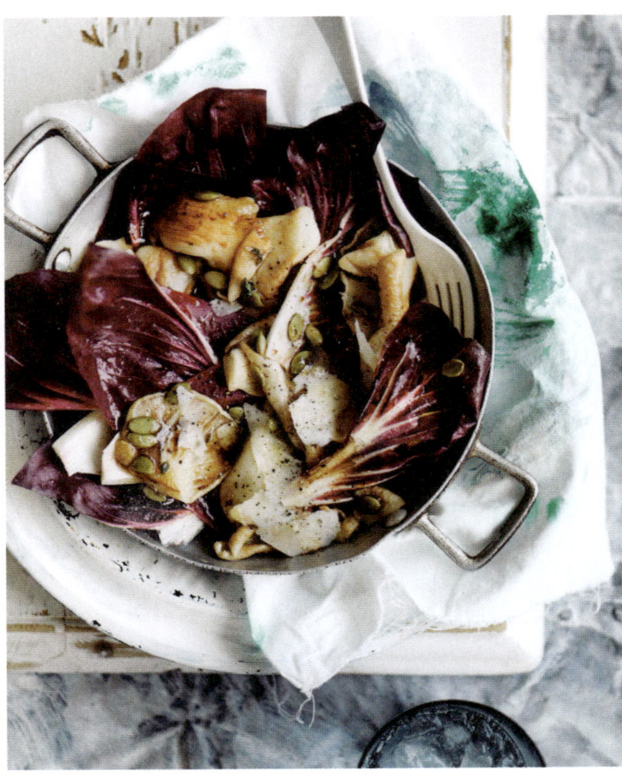

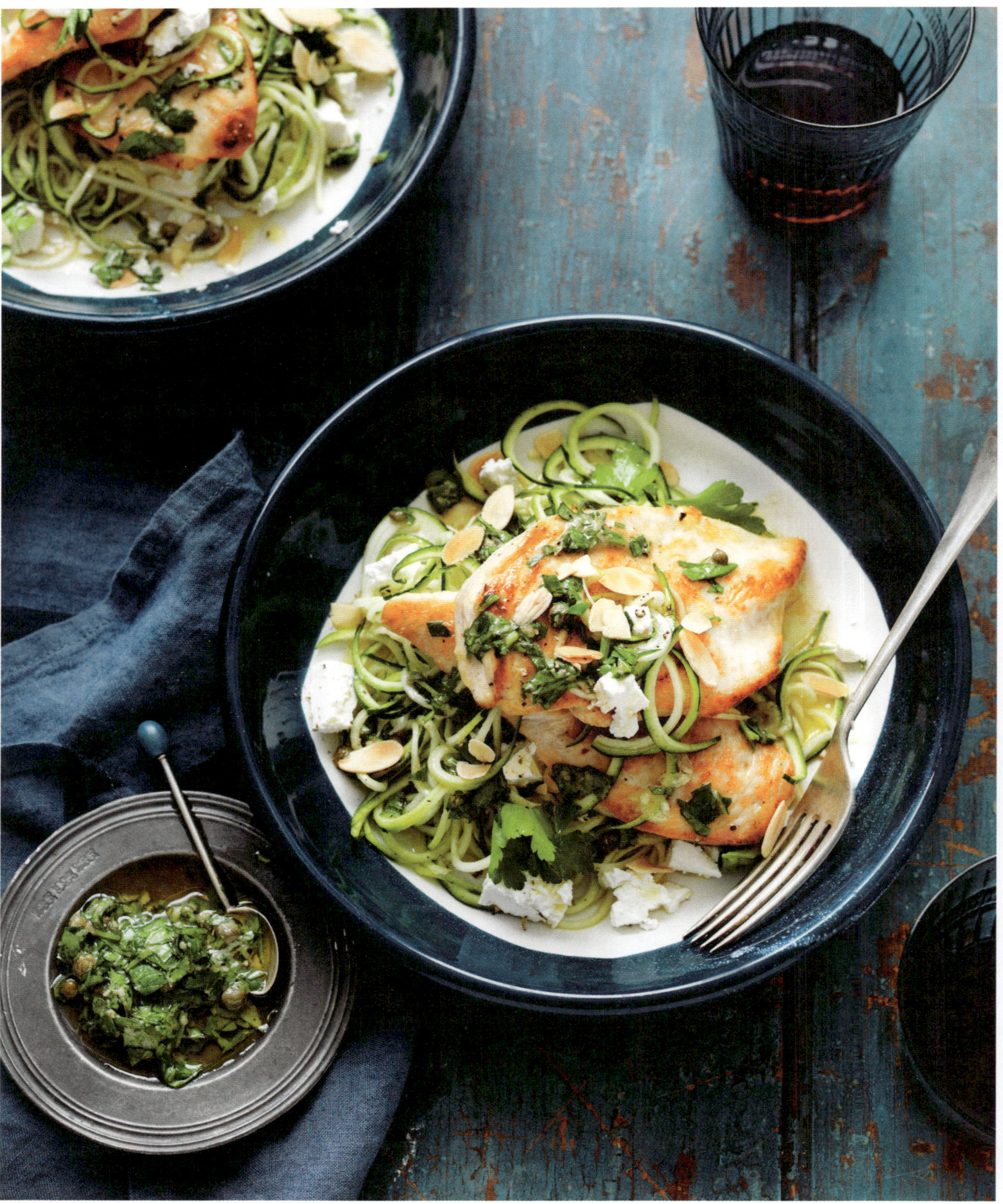

Chicken with zucchini "noodles," feta cheese, and salsa verde

PREP + COOK TIME **35 MINUTES** | SERVES **4**

While to a true Italian, these zucchini "noodles" may seem like heresy, they are a great alternative to pasta when you are looking to have a light summer meal. They also help to increase your vegetable consumption and lower your overall calorie intake.

4 chicken breasts (about 2lb [800g]), trimmed and halved horizontally

1 tbsp olive oil

3 medium zucchini

1/3 cup sliced almonds, toasted

1/2 cup feta cheese, crumbled

1/4 cup fresh Italian parsley leaves

salsa verde

1/2 cup fresh Italian parsley, roughly chopped

1/4 cup fresh basil, roughly chopped

1 garlic clove, crushed

2 tsp nonpareil capers, drained

1 tsp Dijon mustard

1/4 cup olive oil

2 tsp red wine vinegar

salt and freshly ground black pepper

1. Season the chicken on both sides with salt and pepper. Heat the olive oil in a large skillet over medium-high heat; cook the chicken, in batches, for 4 minutes on each side or until browned and cooked through. Transfer to a plate; let stand, covered loosely with foil.
2. Meanwhile, using a vegetable spiralizer (see tip), cut the zucchini into noodles. Set aside.
3. Make the salsa verde. Combine the herbs, garlic, and capers in a small bowl; whisk in the mustard, olive oil, and vinegar until thickened. Season with salt and pepper to taste.
4. Place the zucchini noodles on each plate. Top with a chicken breast and spoonfuls of the salsa verde, the almonds, feta cheese, and parsley. Serve with the remaining salsa verde.

TIP

A spiralizer is a kitchen gadget that cuts vegetables into long thin spirals. If you don't have one, you can use a mandoline or V-slicer to create thin ribbons.

Grilled vegetable and pepper relish paninis

VEGETARIAN | PREP + COOK TIME **50 MINUTES + COOLING** | SERVES **4**

These sandwiches pack a punch in terms of flavors, with the smoky taste of the grill, the umami of the pesto—rich with Parmesan cheese—and the bite of the pepper relish. You can make this relish in advance and refrigerate it in an airtight container for up to a week.

1 large eggplant, cut into ½in (1cm) slices
½lb (200g) pattypan squash, cut into ½in (1cm) slices
1 butternut squash (about ½lb [200g]), peeled, halved, seeds and strings discarded, and thinly sliced
cooking spray
salt and freshly ground black pepper
4 mini baguette rolls, halved lengthways
⅓ cup pesto
⅓ cup soft ricotta cheese
½ cup arugula

pepper relish
1 tbsp olive oil
1 small onion, finely chopped
1 garlic clove, crushed
1 tsp ground cumin
½ tsp chili powder
2 red bell peppers, seeded and roughly chopped
2 yellow bell peppers, seeded and roughly chopped
2 tbsp brown sugar
2 tbsp red wine vinegar

1. Make the pepper relish. Heat the olive oil in a medium frying pan over medium heat. Add the onion, garlic, and spices; cook, covered, for 5 minutes. Add bell peppers; cook, covered, stirring occasionally, for 20 minutes or until soft. Stir in sugar and vinegar; cook until syrupy. Cool.
2. Meanwhile, spray the eggplant, pattypan squash, and butternut squash with oil; season with salt and pepper. Cook the vegetables, in batches, on a heated grill (barbecue) or ridged grill plate over medium-high heat for 3 minutes each side or until browned and tender.
3. Spread each roll with 1 tbsp of the pesto and 1 tbsp of ricotta cheese; top evenly with the vegetables, relish, and arugula.

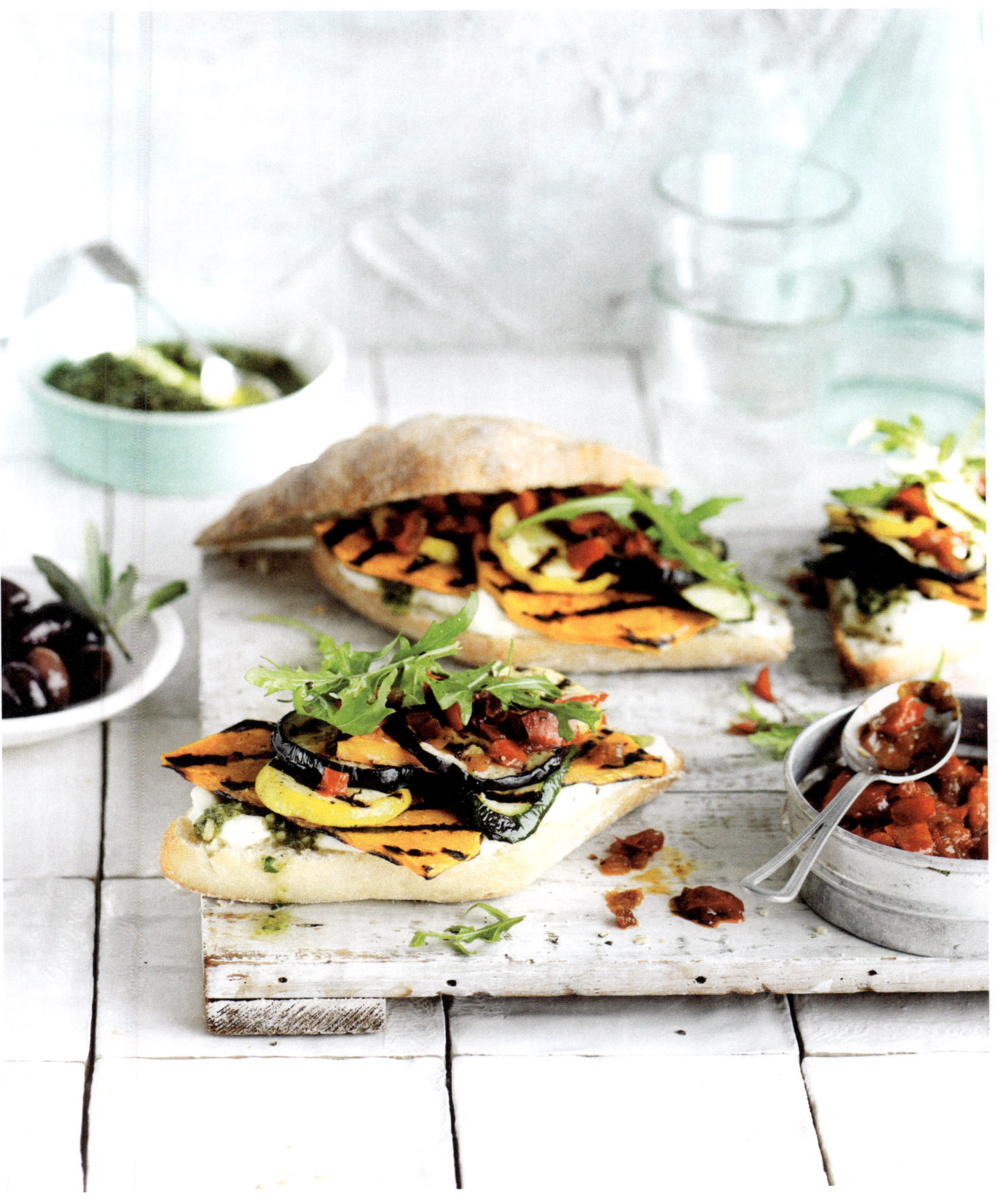

Roasted sumac chicken with baby vegetables

PREP + COOK TIME **1 HOUR 15 MINUTES** | SERVES **4**

This roast chicken makes the perfect family dinner, with any leftovers great for salads or sandwiches the next day. Sumac is a purple-red, astringent spice ground from berries growing on shrubs that flourish wild around the Mediterranean; it adds a tart, lemony flavor to dips and dressings, and goes well with barbecued meats.

2 tbsp butter, softened
1 tbsp sumac
1 whole chicken, 4–5lb (1.8–2.2kg)
salt and freshly ground black pepper
1lb (450g) small beets, trimmed
1 lb (450g) rainbow carrots, peeled, trimmed
1 tbsp olive oil
½ cup fresh mint leaves, to garnish
4oz (100g) feta cheese, crumbled, to garnish
2 tbsp pistachio dukkah, to garnish (see tip)

1 Preheat oven to 350°F (180°C).

2 Combine the butter and sumac in a small bowl. Rub the sumac butter all over the outside of the chicken; season with salt and pepper. Tie chicken legs together with kitchen string; place in a large roasting pan. Wrap the beets individually in foil; add to the pan with the chicken. Roast for 30 minutes.

3 Baste chicken with the pan juices. Toss the carrots in olive oil; season with salt and pepper and add to the roasting pan. Roast for 35 more minutes or until the chicken reaches an internal temperature of 165°F (80°C) and skin is golden brown. Cover the chicken loosely with foil; let stand for 10 minutes.

4 Meanwhile, peel the beets and cut in half. Return them to the roasting pan.

5 Serve the roast chicken and vegetables topped with the mint, feta cheese, and dukkah.

TIP

Dukkah is a nut-seed blend popular in North Africa and the Middle East. You can find it at international markets or gourmet grocery stores.

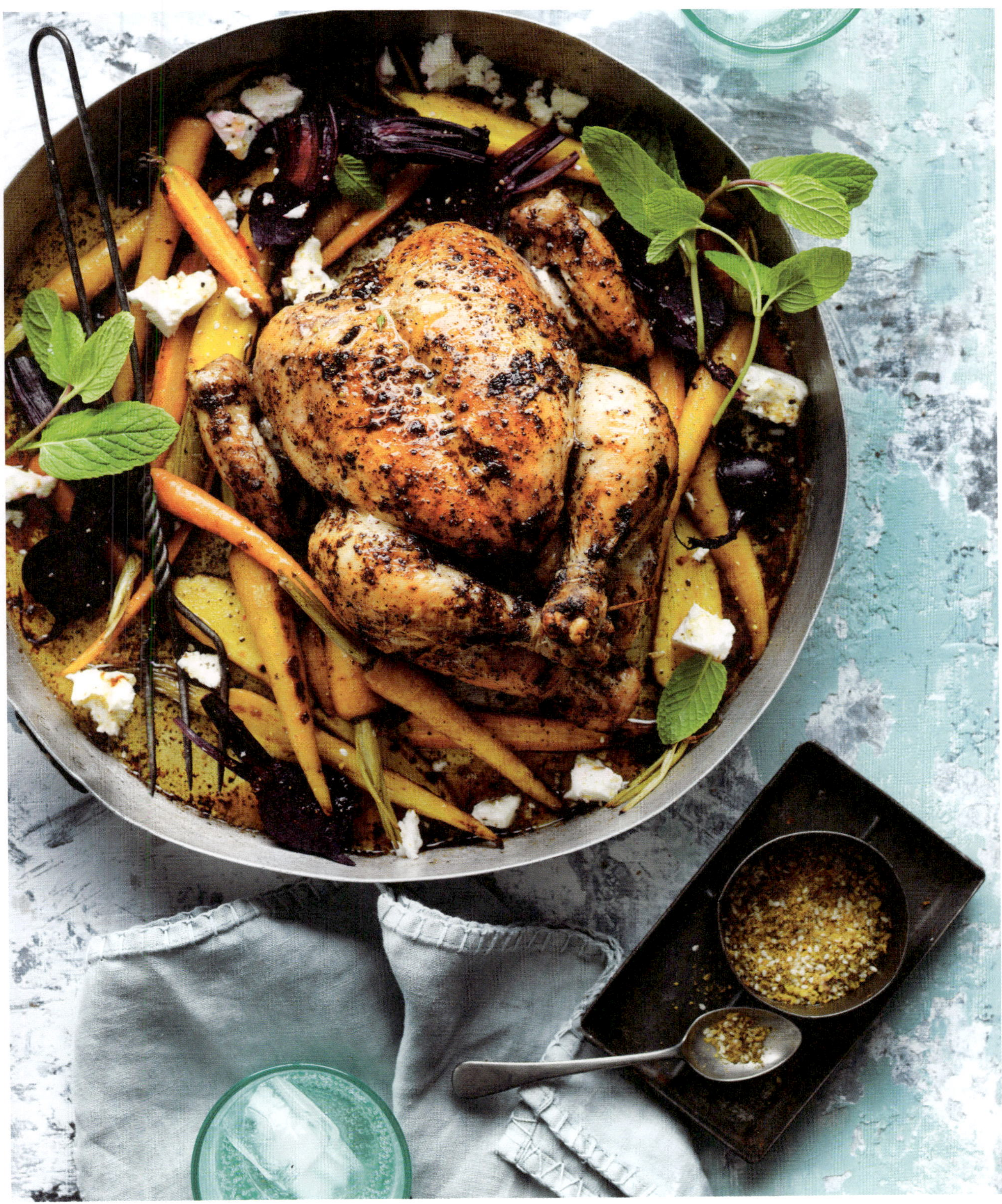

Pea and barley risotto with garlic shrimp

PREP + COOK TIME **1 HOUR** | SERVES **4**

Risotto is traditionally made using short-grain rice such as carnaroli or arborio, but here we use barley, a nutritious cereal grain that is higher in fiber than processed white rice. Soluble fiber has been shown to lower levels of blood cholesterol, while also improving the regulation of blood sugar. However, unlike rice, barley is not gluten-free.

¼ cup olive oil, divided
1 fresh long red chile, finely chopped
4 garlic cloves, finely chopped, divided
2 shallots, finely chopped
1 cup pearl barley
4 cups chicken stock
1 tbsp finely grated lemon zest
½ cup frozen peas
1 cup sugar snap peas, trimmed, halved lengthwise
salt and freshly ground black pepper
1lb (400g) uncooked shrimp
extra finely grated lemon zest, to garnish

1 Heat 1 tbsp of olive oil in a large heavy-bottomed saucepan over low-medium heat, add the chile, half the garlic, and the shallots; cook, stirring, for 3 minutes or until tender. Add the barley; cook, stirring, for 2 minutes or until lightly toasted. Add 2 cups of the stock; bring to a boil. Reduce heat to low; cook, covered, stirring occasionally, for 18 minutes or until the liquid has been absorbed. Add the remaining stock and 1 cup water; cook, stirring occasionally, for 18 more minutes or until most of the liquid has been absorbed. Add the lemon zest, peas, and sugar snap peas; cook, stirring, for 3 minutes or until the vegetables are tender. Season with salt and pepper to taste.

2 Meanwhile, peel and devein the shrimp, leaving the tails intact. Heat the remaining olive oil in a medium skillet over high heat; cook the shrimp and the remaining garlic, stirring, for 3–5 minutes or until shrimp are just cooked. Season with salt and pepper.

3 Divide the risotto among four bowls; top with the shrimp and extra lemon zest.

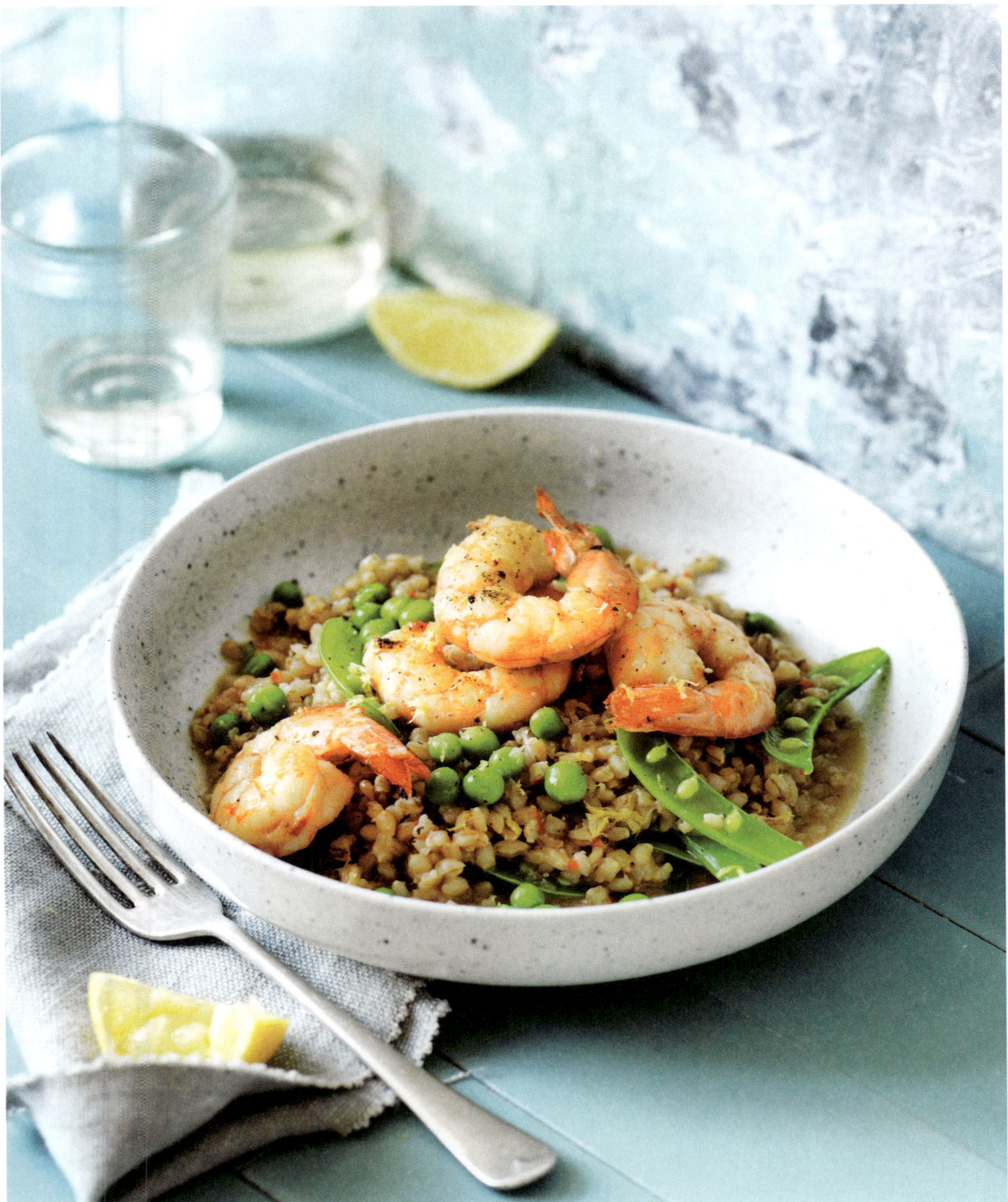

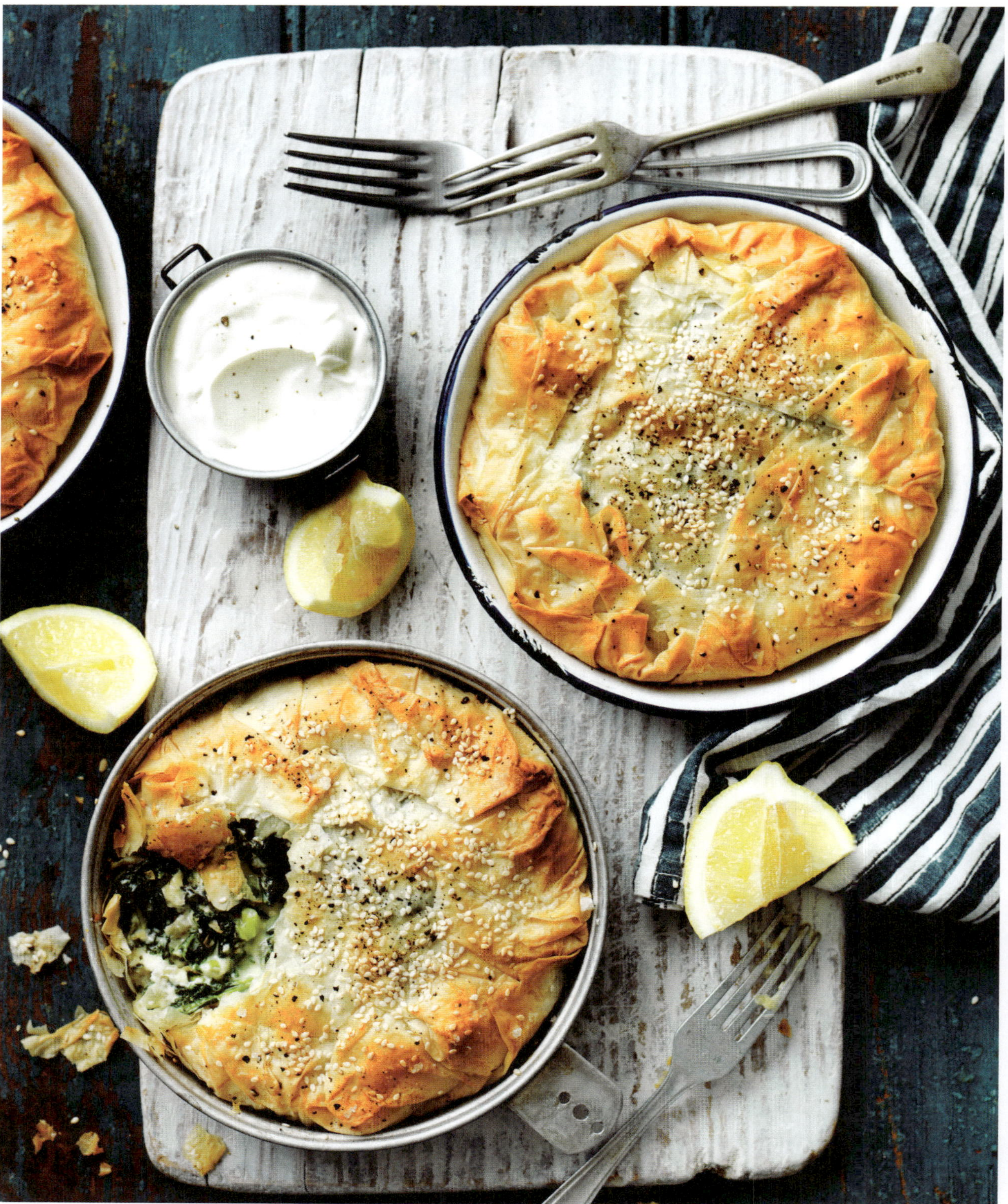

Kale and spinach spanakopitas

VEGETARIAN | PREP + COOK TIME **1 HOUR 45 MINUTES** | MAKES **6**

Spanakopita is known the world over. A family favorite, this phyllo-crusted pie is eaten across all the regions of Greece. In rural areas the greens are often a mixture of spinach with leek, chard, or sorrel. Here we also add the superfood kale, a nutritious leafy cabbage, for an extra nutrient boost. Serve with Greek yogurt, if you like.

1lb (450g) Swiss chard
3/4 lb (350g) curly kale (approximately 1 bunch)
2 tbsp olive oil, divided
14oz (400g) feta cheese, crumbled
10 spring onions, finely chopped
1/2 cup fresh dill, finely chopped
3/4 cup fresh Italian parsley, finely chopped
2 tsp finely grated lemon zest
1/4 cup lemon juice
3 eggs, lightly beaten
freshly ground black pepper
6 tbsp butter, melted
16 sheets frozen phyllo dough, 14 x 18in (36 x 46cm)
2 tsp sesame seeds
lemon wedges, for serving

TIP

You can make this pie in advance through the end of step 5. Simply cover and refrigerate until you're ready to bake.

1 Preheat oven to 350°F (180°C).

2 Remove the chard leaves from each stalk, retaining the stalks. Finely chop the chard leaves. Trim the stalks 2in (5cm) from the bottom and finely chop the stalks, Separately, trim and finely chop the kale.

3 Heat a large skillet over medium-high heat; add 1 tbsp of olive oil and cook the chard stems, stirring occasionally, for 10 minutes or until softened. Drain well; transfer to a large bowl. Add the chopped chard and kale leaves to the pan; cook for 2 minutes or until wilted. Drain well; add to the bowl with the stems. When cool enough to handle, squeeze excess water from the greens mixture.

4 In a large bow, combine the sautéed greens, feta cheese, green onion, herbs, lemon zest, lemon juice, and eggs; season with freshly ground black pepper.

5 Brush the melted butter on the inside of two 9in (23cm) cake pans or pie dishes. Working with a damp towel over your phyllo dough, lift one sheet and place it in the center of the pan with the edges overhanging. Brush the center of the pastry with melted butter and repeat with next sheet of pastry, laying it across at a 90° angle. Place 8 layers of pastry total in each pan, adjusting the angle for each layer so pastry overhangs the entire pan. Repeat with second pan. Divide the vegetable mixture between each pan. Then, working with the remaining melted butter, fold the pastry flaps over the filling, brushing butter between the overlapping layers. You can scrunch any extra pastry as you fold. Brush the top of each pie with melted butter. Sprinkle with sesame seeds.

6 Sprinkle a little water over each pie; this will prevent the pastry from burning. Bake for 35–40 minutes or until golden. Serve with lemon wedges.

Beef souvlaki with fennel and garlic yogurt

PREP + COOK TIME **40 MINUTES + REFRIGERATION** | SERVES **4**

There is something so comforting in these small pieces of meat cooked on skewers, with their smoky, grilled flavor and the pleasure of eating with your hands. You can use bamboo or metal skewers instead of rosemary skewers, if you like.

1 medium lemon
2 tbsp olive oil
1/3 cup dry white wine
1 tbsp fresh rosemary, finely chopped
1 bay leaf, torn
2 garlic cloves, crushed
salt and freshly ground black pepper
2lb (1kg) beef sirloin, tri-tip, or strip steak, cut into 1 1/2in (4cm) pieces
8 fresh rosemary stalks
grilled pita bread, for serving

fennel salad

2 medium fennel bulbs
2 tbsp olive oil
1 tbsp red wine vinegar
1/2 cup mixed pitted olives

garlic yogurt

1 cup Greek yogurt
2 garlic cloves, crushed

1. Zest the entire lemon and set lemon zest aside. Roughly chop the lemon flesh and the remaining rind.
2. In a large nonreactive bowl, combine the olive oil, lemon zest and chopped lemon, wine, chopped rosemary, torn bay leaf, and garlic; season with salt and pepper. Add the beef, toss to coat in the mixture. Cover; refrigerate for 1 hour or overnight.
3. To make the fennel salad, trim the base of the fennel bulbs; reserve the fronds. Using a mandoline or V-slicer, thinly slice the fennel lengthwise; place in a bowl of iced water. Drain well, lightly pat dry. Finely chop the fennel fronds. Place the fennel, half the reserved fennel fronds, olive oil, vinegar, and olives in a medium bowl; toss well to combine. Season with salt and pepper to taste.
4. To make the garlic yogurt, place the ingredients in a small bowl with the remaining fennel fronds; stir to combine. Season with salt and pepper to taste.
5. Bring the beef to room temperature. Evenly thread the beef onto the rosemary stalks.
6. Cook the skewers on a heated grill (barbecue) or ridged grill pan over medium-high heat, turning occasionally, for 5 minutes for medium rare, or until cooked as desired.
7. Serve skewers with the grilled pita, fennel salad, and garlic yogurt.

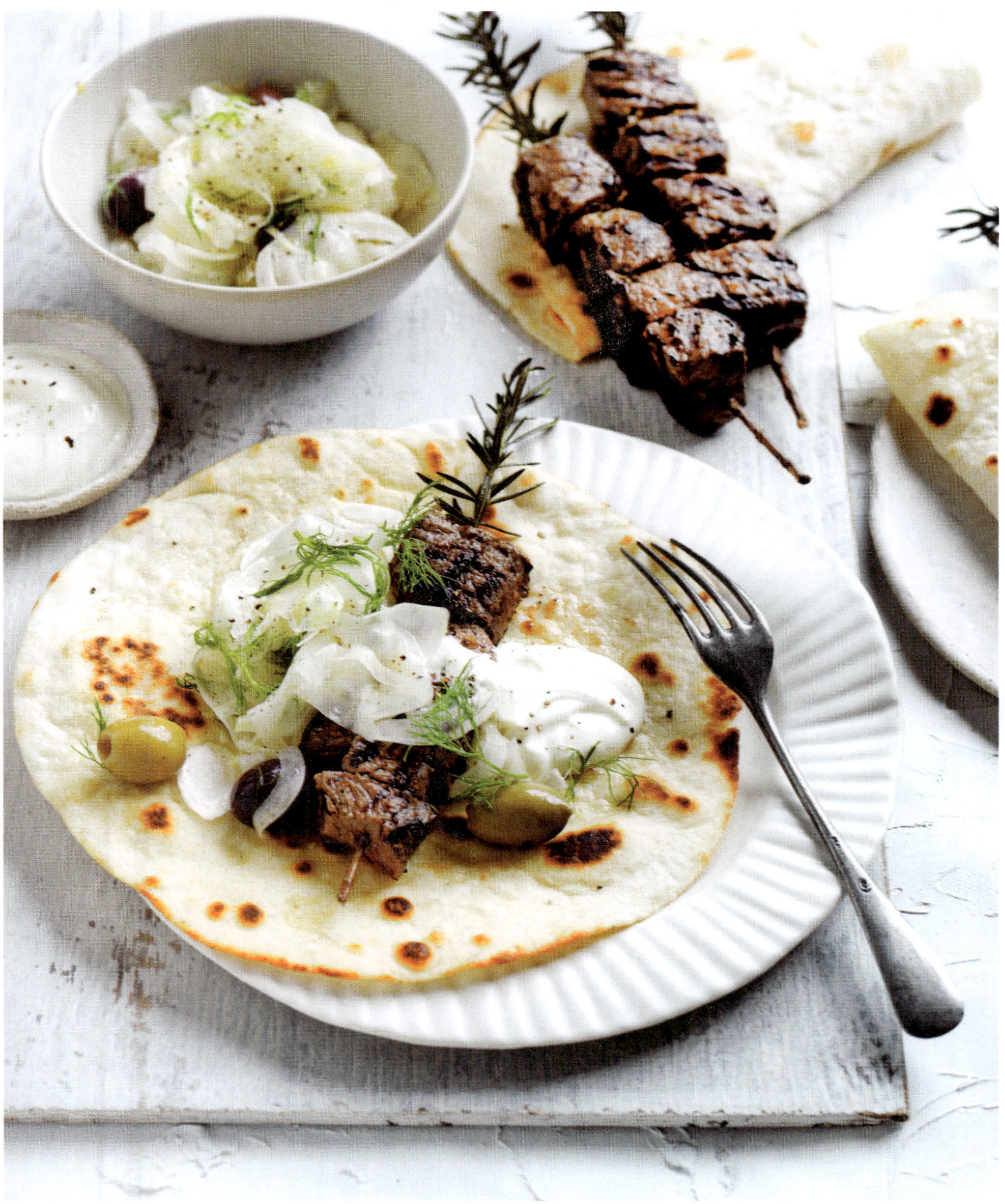

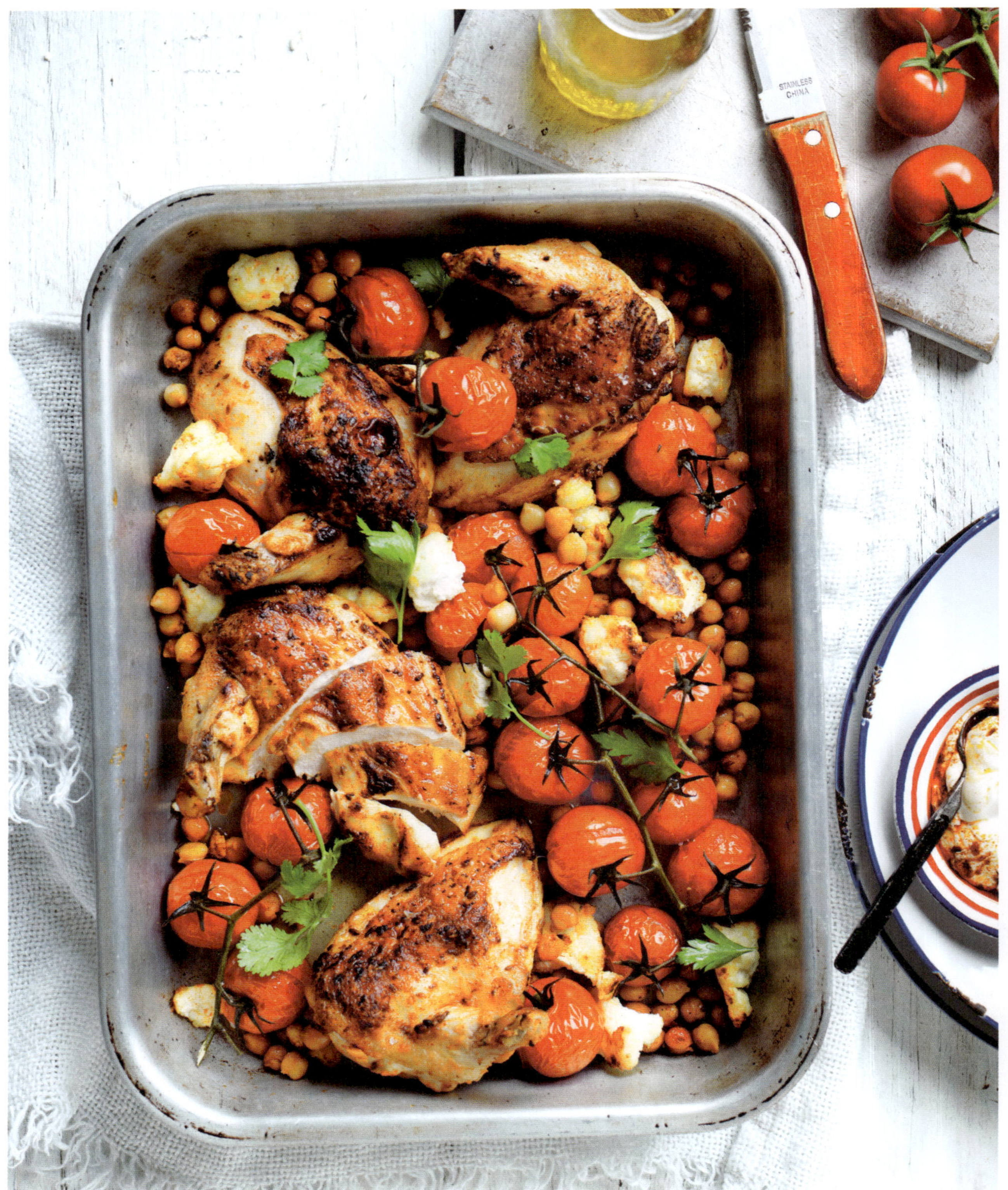
STAINLESS
CHINA

Paprika and cumin spiced roast chicken with chickpeas

PREP + COOK TIME **45 MINUTES** | SERVES **4**

Paprika is a ground spice made from dried sweet red peppers, with grades including sweet, mild, smoked, and hot. The hotter types are usually combined with ground chile peppers or cayenne pepper. Originating in central Mexico, paprika was brought to Spain in the 16th century, and is often used to add color, as well as flavor, to many types of dishes.

4 garlic cloves, crushed
1 tbsp smoked paprika
1 tsp cumin seeds
$1/2$ cup olive oil, divided
$1/2$ cup Greek yogurt
salt and freshly ground black pepper
4 x $1/2$ lb (200g) airline chicken breasts (see tip)
1 x 15oz (400g) can chickpeas, drained, rinsed
10oz (285g) cherry tomatoes
$3/4$ cup firm ricotta cheese, broken into large chunks
$1/4$ cup cilantro sprigs, to garnish
$1/4$ cup fresh Italian parsley leaves, to garnish

1. Preheat oven to 475°F (240°C).
2. Combine the garlic, paprika, cumin, and $1/3$ cup of olive oil in a small bowl. Place 2 tsp of this spice oil mixture in another bowl. Set aside. Combine the spiced oil with the yogurt; season with salt and pepper. Cover the yogurt mixture; refrigerate until required.
3. Rub 2 tbsp of the reserved spice oil mixture over the chicken; season with salt and pepper. Heat the remaining olive oil in a large frying pan over high heat; cook the chicken for 2 minutes each side or until browned. Transfer chicken to a deep roasting pan. Roast the chicken in the oven for 10 minutes.
4. Reduce oven to 400°F (200°C). Combine the chickpeas, tomatoes, ricotta cheese, and remaining spice oil mixture in a large bowl. Spoon the chickpea mixture around the chicken in the pan; season with salt and pepper. Roast for another 15 minutes or until the chicken is cooked to an internal temperature of 165°F (74°C).
5. Serve the chicken and chickpea mixture with the yogurt sauce, sprinkled with cilantro and parsley.

TIP

Airline chicken, also called chicken supremes, is a cut that includes the chicken breast with the wing bone still attached. The skin will usually be on. If your butcher doesn't have them, order them in advance or substitute for a bone-in chicken breast.

Za'atar fish with bulgur salad

PESCATARIAN | PREP + COOK TIME **30 MINUTES + STANDING** | SERVES **4**

Spices and herbs are integral to a Mediterranean diet, adding flavor to dishes without fat or sugar. Some of the most common spices found in Mediterranean cuisine include cumin, saffron, sumac, and za'atar. Common herbs of the region, used both in their fresh and dried forms, include oregano, sage, coriander (cilantro), parsley, thyme, basil, and rosemary.

1 tbsp olive oil
1½ tbsp za'atar (see tips)
4 x 6oz (180g) boneless white fish filets (see tips)
salt and freshly ground black pepper

bulgur salad
1 medium red onion, thinly sliced
1 cup fresh Italian parsley
1 tbsp fresh thyme leaves
4 Roma tomatoes, roughly chopped
½ cup radishes, thinly sliced
2 cups arugula
¼ cup bulgur
1 tsp ground sumac
2 tbsp lemon juice
¼ cup olive oil

1. Make the bulgur salad. Combine the ingredients in a large bowl; season with salt and pepper to taste. Let stand for 15 minutes or until the bulgur is softened.
2. Combine the olive oil, za'atar, and fish in a large bowl; season with salt and pepper. Cook the fish in a 9in (23cm) skillet or on a heated grill (barbecue) or ridged grill pan over medium-high heat for 2 minutes on each side, or until browned and cooked through.
3. Serve the fish with the bulgur salad.

TIPS

- Za'atar is available in major supermarkets and Middle Eastern food stores.
- This recipe is perfect with light white fish like Mediterranean sea bass, branzino, trout, or even tilapia. For something more substantial, try salmon.

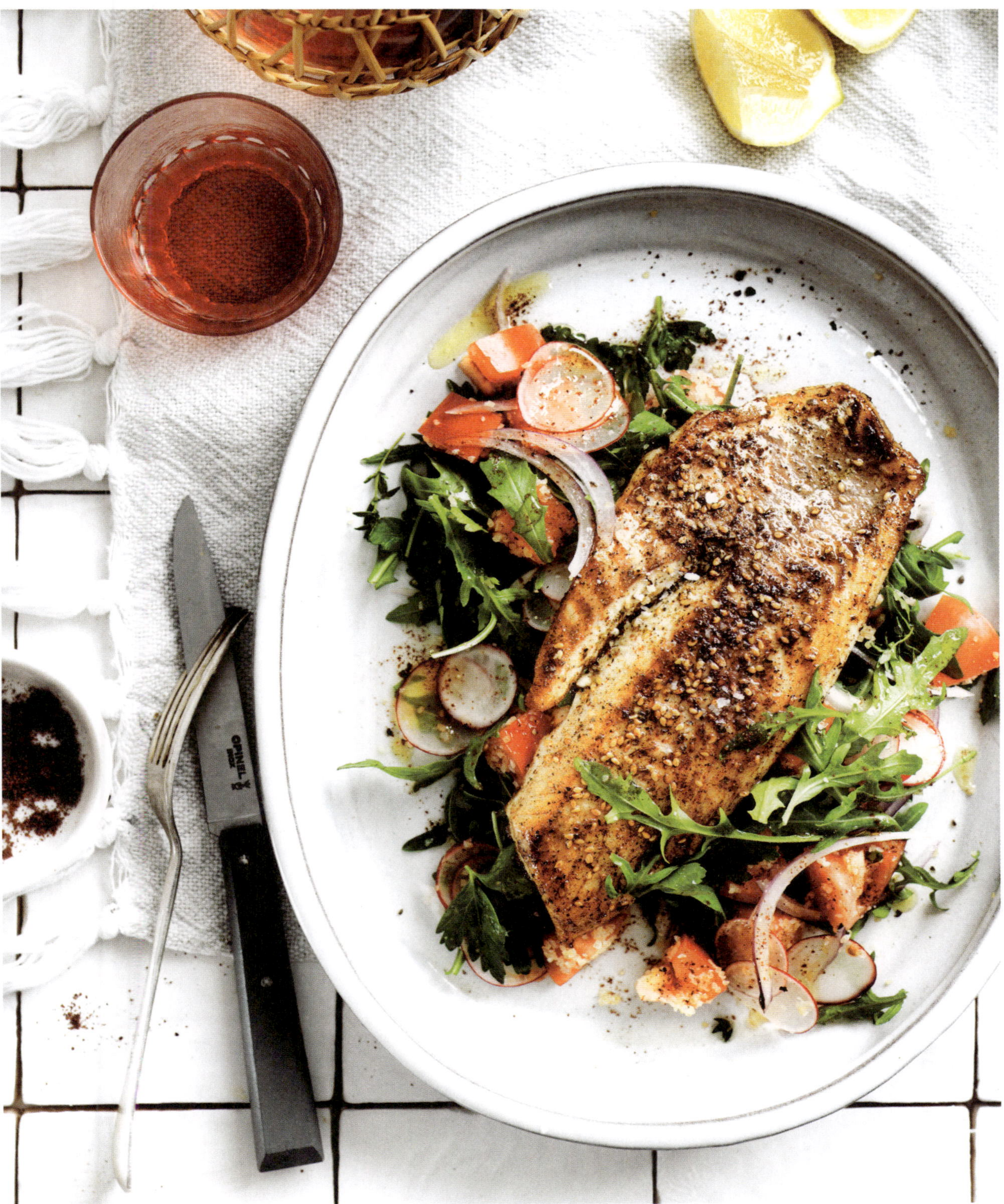
OPINEL

Butternut squash and goat cheese lasagna

VEGETARIAN | PREP + COOK TIME **3 HOURS** | SERVES **10**

Though it's an Italian staple, lasagna originated in Ancient Greece—the word "lasagna" is derived from the Greek word *laganon*, which is the first known form of pasta. The ingredients Italians use in their recipe will depend on the part of Italy their family came from, but this healthy, fresh veggie version provides a lighter take on the classic dish.

3–4 large butternut squash (4½–5lb [3.4kg]), halved lengthways
2 tbsp olive oil, divided
salt and freshly ground black pepper
4 medium leeks, thinly sliced
4 garlic cloves, crushed
½ tsp ground nutmeg
4 cups firm ricotta cheese
3 egg yolks
1 tsp finely grated lemon zest
1¼ cups finely grated Parmesan cheese
1 cup light cream
¼ cup fresh sage leaves, finely chopped
1½ tbsp fresh chives, finely chopped
1 x 1lb (450g) box dried wavy lasagna sheets, prepared according to package instructions
5oz (150g) soft goat cheese, crumbled

arugula and pumpkin seed salad
2 tsp lemon juice
1 tsp whole-grain mustard
1½ tbsp olive oil
4 cups arugula
¼ cup pumpkin seeds, toasted

1. Preheat oven to 400°F (200°C). Line two baking sheets with parchment paper.
2. Divide the squash halves, skin-side up, between two large baking sheets; brush each half with 1 tbsp of olive oil. Season with salt and pepper. Cover with foil; bake for 30–40 minutes or until very tender. Let cool. Remove the seeds, then peel away skin. Add the squash to the bowl of a food processor and pulse until smooth. Set aside.
3. Heat the remaining olive oil in a large saucepan over medium heat; cook the leeks and garlic, stirring occasionally, for 10 minutes or until soft. Combine the leek mixture, puréed squash, and nutmeg. Season with salt and pepper to taste. Set aside.
4. In a food processor, process ricotta cheese, egg yolks, and lemon zest in batches until smooth. Add 1 cup of Parmesan cheese and cream, pulse until just combined. Stir in herbs. Season with salt and pepper.
5. Oil a 9 x 13in (23 x 33cm) ovenproof baking dish. Place a layer of lasagna noodles in the bottom of the dish. Spoon a third of the ricotta cheese mixture over the noodles, smoothing to the edges. Top with half of the squash mixture. Add another layer of lasagna noodles, then another third of the ricotta mixture, and the remaining half of the squash mixture. Top with the remaining lasagna noodles and the remaining ricotta mixture. Sprinkle with the goat cheese and the remaining Parmesan cheese. Cover with a layer of aluminum foil.
6. Bake lasagna for 50 minutes. Remove foil and paper; bake for 15 more minutes or until golden and hot. Let stand for 10 minutes.
7. Meanwhile, to make the arugula and pumpkin seed salad, combine the lemon juice, mustard, and olive oil in a large bowl; season with salt and pepper to taste. Add the arugula and pumpkin seeds; toss gently to combine. Serve the lasagna with the salad.

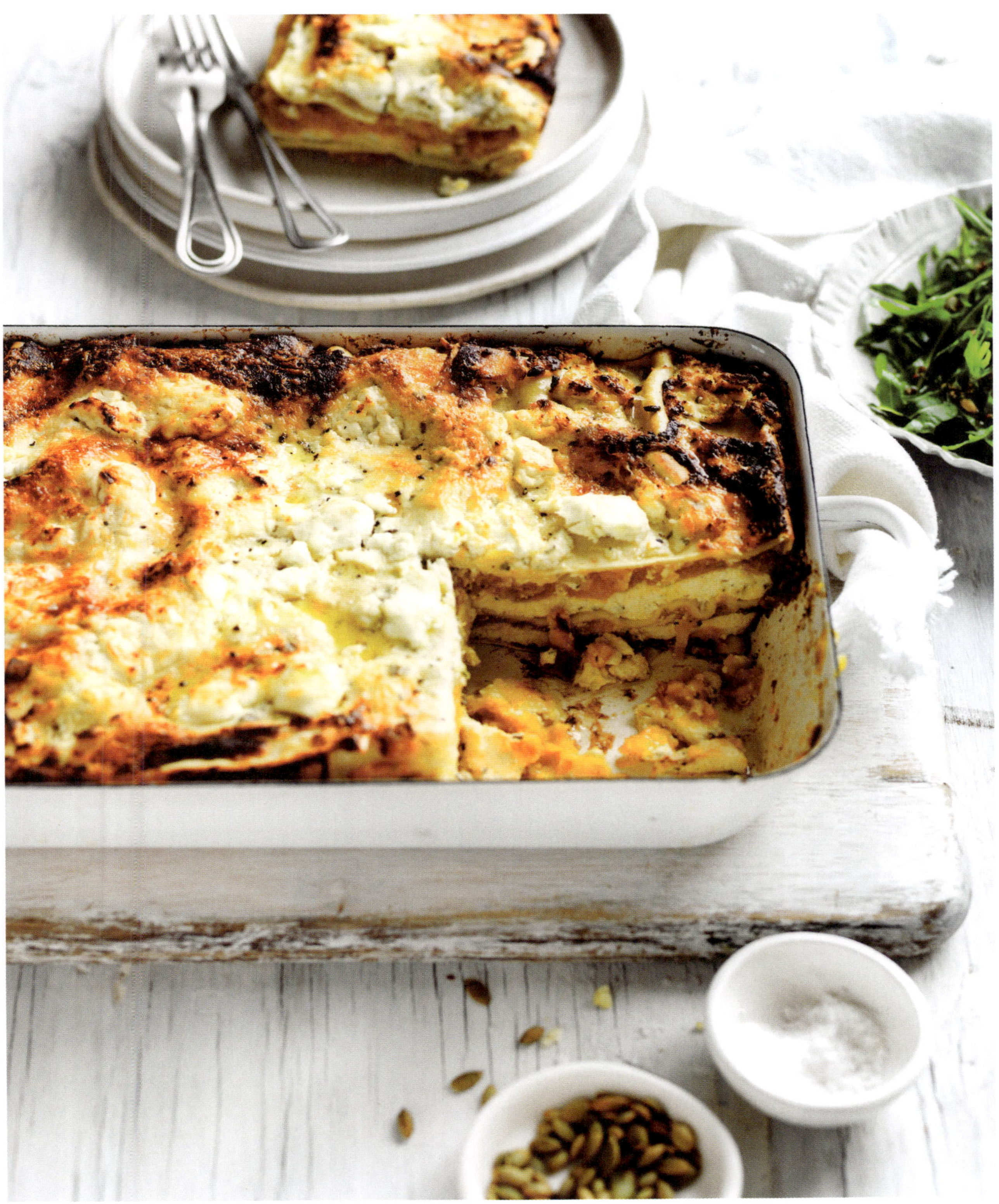

Greek roast leg of lamb with lemon potatoes and skordalia

PREP + COOK TIME **4 HOURS 45 MINUTES + REFRIGERATION** | SERVES **4**

Skordalia is a classic Greek accompaniment to meat—a kind of dip or spread—made from either potato or bread pureed with garlic, olive oil, lemon juice or vinegar, herbs, and, occasionally, ground nuts. To serve, sprinkle the roast lamb with extra fresh lemon thyme sprigs, if you like.

2 garlic cloves, crushed
½ cup lemon juice
2 tbsp olive oil
1 tbsp fresh oregano leaves
1 tsp fresh lemon thyme leaves
4–5lb (2kg) leg of lamb, bone in
lemon wedges, for serving

skordalia

1 medium russet potato, peeled, quartered
3 garlic cloves, peeled and roughly chopped
1 tbsp lemon juice
1 tbsp white wine vinegar
⅓ cup olive oil

lemon potatoes

2lb (1kg) small red or white potatoes
1 medium lemon, zest peeled with a vegetable peeler into 6 wide strips
2 tbsp lemon juice
2 tbsp olive oil
salt and freshly ground black pepper

1. Combine the garlic, lemon juice, olive oil, oregano, and thyme leaves in a large nonreactive bowl; add the lamb, turn to coat in the mixture. Cover; refrigerate for 3 hours or overnight.
2. Preheat oven to 325°F (160°C).
3. Place the marinated lamb in a large roasting pan; roast for 3½ hours.
4. Meanwhile, to make the skordalia, boil, steam, or microwave the potato until tender; drain. Push the potato through a ricer or fine sieve into a medium bowl; let cool for 10 minutes. Add the garlic, lemon juice, vinegar, and 2 tbsp water to the potato; stir until well combined. Place the potato mixture in a blender or food processor; with the processor running, gradually add the olive oil in a thin, steady stream, blending only until the skordalia thickens (do not overmix or the sauce will become gluey). Stir in 1 tbsp warm water.
5. To make the lemon potatoes, combine the potatoes, lemon zest, lemon juice, and olive oil in a large bowl; season with salt and pepper. Place, in a single layer, on a baking sheet lined with parchment paper.
6. Put the baking sheet with the lemon potatoes in the oven; roast alongside the lamb for the last 30 minutes of lamb cooking time.
7. Remove the lamb from the oven; let stand, covered loosely with foil.
8. Increase oven to 450°F (220°C); roast the potatoes 20 additional minutes or until golden, stirring twice.
9. Serve the roast lamb with the lemon potatoes, skordalia, and lemon wedges.

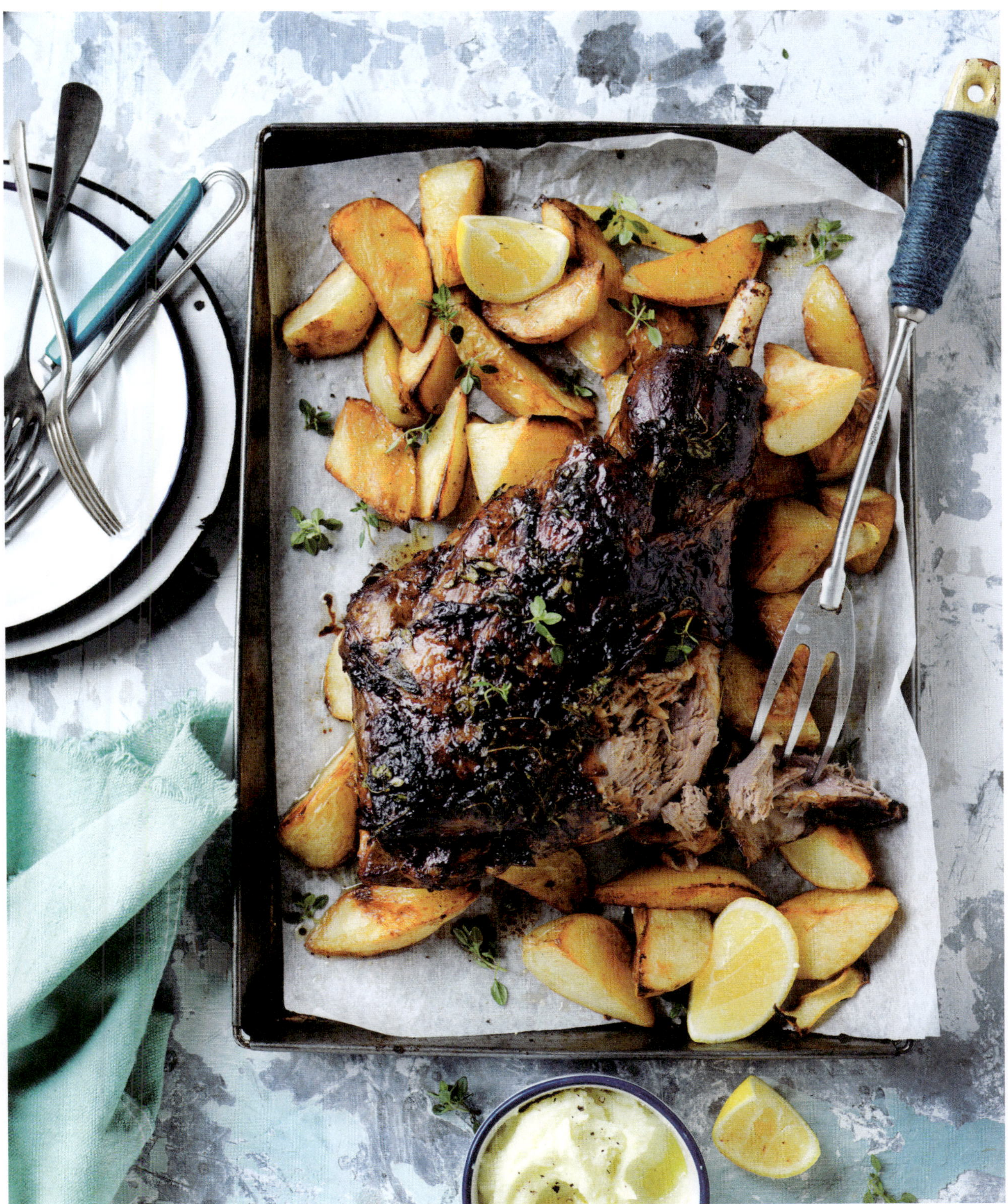

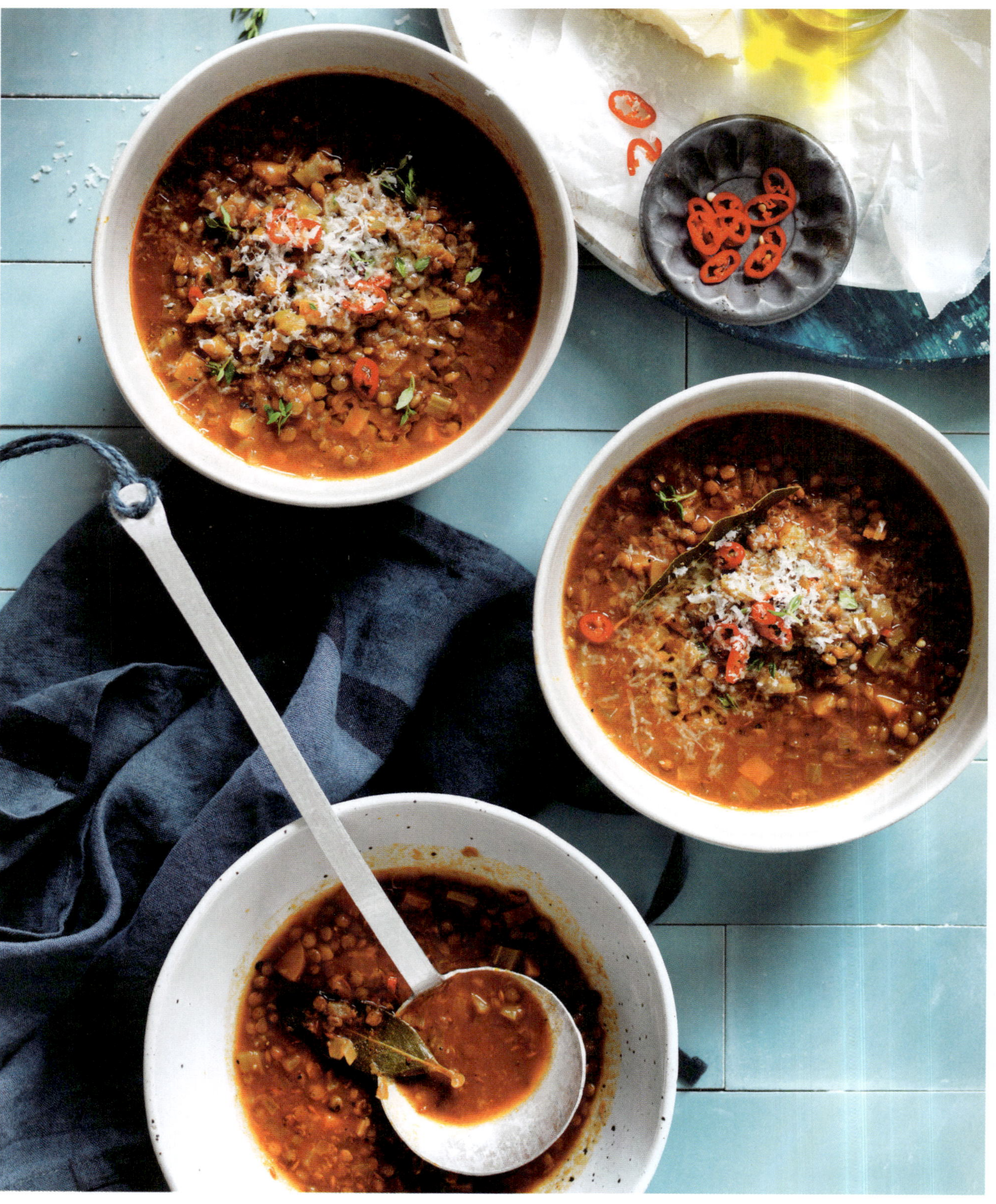

Hearty Italian lentil and vegetable soup

VEGETARIAN | PREP + COOK TIME **50 MINUTES** | SERVES **4**

While meaty stews are often the comfort food of choice when the weather gets chilly, a big bowl of lentil soup is a great vegetarian substitute. After soybeans, lentils have the second-highest ratio of protein per kilojoules of any legume, and they are rich in folate, vitamin B6, and iron.

1 tbsp olive oil
1 medium onion, finely chopped
3 garlic cloves, crushed
2 tsp finely grated fresh ginger
1 tsp cumin seeds, lightly crushed
1 fresh long red chile, finely chopped
1 medium carrot, finely chopped
3 celery stalks, trimmed and finely chopped
2 fresh bay leaves
3 fresh thyme sprigs, plus extra for serving
1¼ cups dried French-style green lentils, rinsed
¼ cup tomato paste
6 cups vegetable stock
1½ tbsp lemon juice
salt and freshly ground black pepper
⅓ cup finely grated Parmesan cheese
1 fresh long red chile, extra, thinly sliced

1. Heat the olive oil in a large pot over medium-high heat; cook the onion, garlic, ginger, cumin, chile, carrot, and celery, stirring, for 10 minutes or until the vegetables are softened.
2. Add the bay leaves, thyme, lentils, tomato paste, and stock, bring to a boil; reduce heat to low. Cook for 20 minutes or until the lentils are tender. Stir in the lemon juice; season with salt and pepper to taste.
3. Ladle the soup into bowls, top with the Parmesan cheese and extra chile. Sprinkle with extra thyme before serving, if you like.

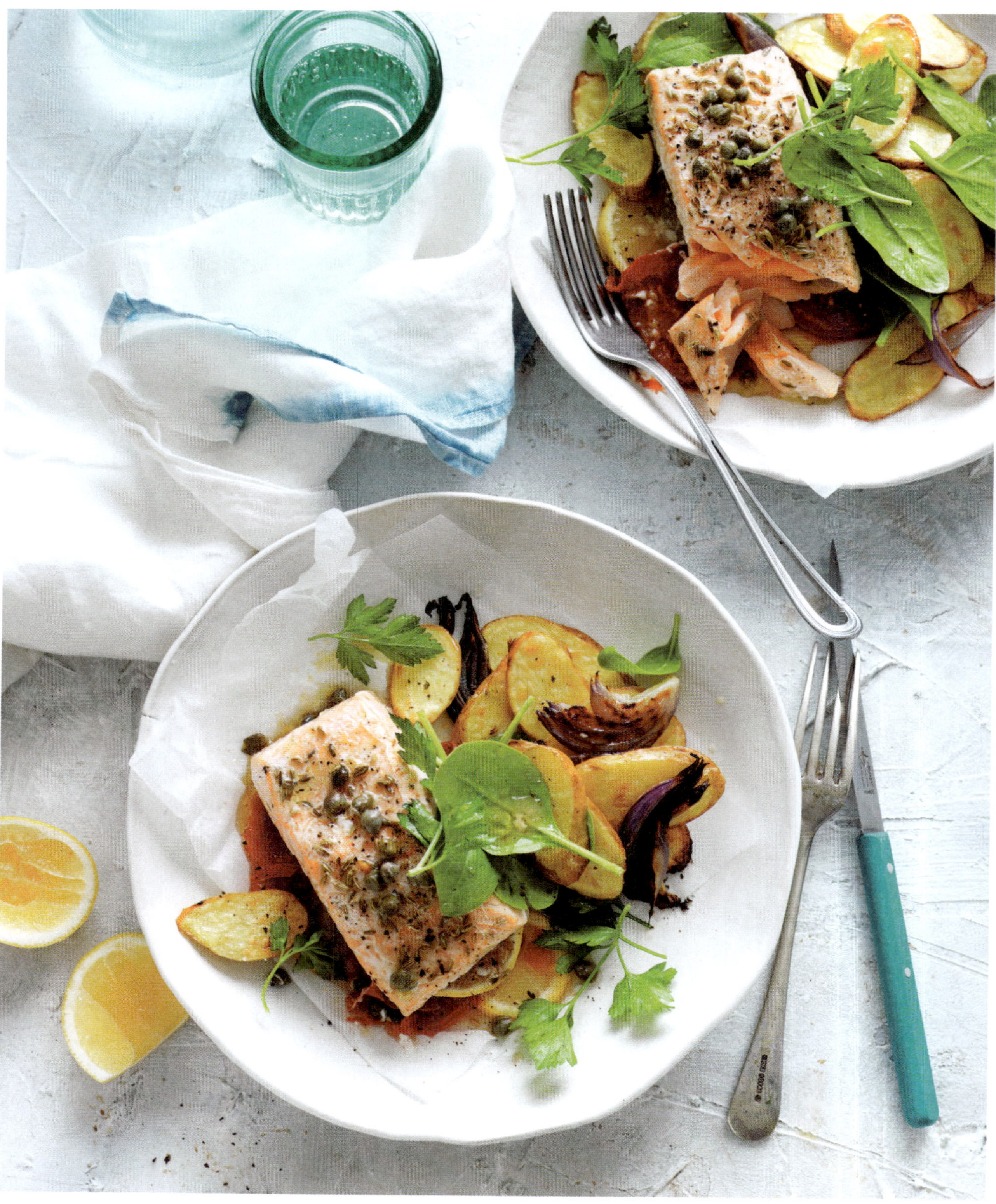

Salmon parcels with fingerling potatoes

PESCATARIAN | PREP + COOK TIME **50 MINUTES** | SERVES **2**

After tuna, salmon might be the most popular fish in the world to eat. Luckily, when baked, pan-fried, or grilled, salmon is also among the most heart-healthy of fish. It is packed with vitamins and minerals, such as B12, vitamin D, and selenium, and is a good source of niacin, omega-3 fatty acids, protein, phosphorus, and potassium.

1lb (300g) fingerling potatoes, thinly sliced
1 small red onion, cut into thin wedges
1 tbsp olive oil, divided
½ medium lemon, thinly sliced
1 medium tomato, thinly sliced
2 x 6oz (180g) salmon fillets, boneless, preferably with skin on
2 tsp nonpareil capers
1 tsp fennel seeds
3 cups spinach leaves
¼ cup fresh Italian parsley leaves

1. Preheat oven to 400°F (200°C). Line a large baking sheet with parchment paper.
2. Combine the potato and onion on the baking sheet; drizzle with ½ tsp olive oil. Roast for 30 minutes or until lightly browned and tender, stirring once or twice while roasting.
3. Meanwhile, stack the lemon and the tomato slices on two pieces of parchment paper 12in (30cm) square. Top with the salmon, capers, and fennel seeds; drizzle with the remaining olive oil. Fold the paper into a parcel to enclose the salmon; twist closed or tie loosely with kitchen twine. Place on a baking sheet. Bake for 8 minutes or until the salmon is cooked as desired.
4. Serve the salmon parcels with the potato and onion; top with spinach and parsley.

TIPS

- Baking the salmon in a parcel locks in all the flavors, juices, and steam to give a moist and flavorful result.
- You could try using firm white fish fillets or even chicken breast instead of salmon, adjusting your cooking times as needed.

Cheese and Swiss chard borek with crunchy seeds

VEGETARIAN | PREP + COOK TIME **1 HOUR 20 MINUTES** | SERVES **6**

Borek are pastry-enclosed treats that are popular in Turkey. Stuffed with cheese, meat, and vegetables, they can take on many forms, offering a crispy, savory start for any meal. This one uses Swiss chard in place of the more traditional spinach, along with cheese and hardy seeds.

1lb (480g) Swiss chard, about 6 ribs
2 tbsp olive oil
5 eggs, divided
2 cups firm ricotta cheese (see tip)
7oz (200g) feta cheese, crumbled
1 cup sour cream
1/2 cup club soda
salt and freshly ground black pepper
10 phyllo dough sheets, 14 x 18in (36 x 46cm)
olive oil cooking spray
1 tsp poppy seeds
1 tbsp sunflower seeds
1 tbsp pumpkin seeds
Greek yogurt, for serving
1 medium lemon, cut into wedges

TIP

Fresh firm ricotta cheese purchased from a cheese counter or specialty shop is best for this recipe.

1. Preheat oven to 350°F (180°C). Line a 9 x 13in (22 x 32cm) ovenproof baking dish with parchment paper extending up over the sides.
2. Trim 1½in (4cm) from the bottom of the Swiss chard stems. Slice the leaves from the stems. Finely chop the leaves. Separately, finely chop the stems.
3. Heat a large skillet over high heat. Add the olive oil. Cook the chopped chard stems for 3 minutes, then add the leaves and cook for 2 minutes more until wilted and tender. When cool, squeeze any excess liquid from the chard leaves and stems. Set aside.
4. Whisk 4 of the eggs in a large bowl until combined. Add the ricotta cheese, feta cheese, sour cream, club soda, and chard, stir to combine; season with salt and pepper.
5. Layer three sheets of phyllo dough in the bottom of the baking dish, spraying with cooking spray between each layer. Let the edges extend up the side of the dish. Keep the remaining sheets covered with baking paper topped with a clean, damp paper towel to prevent them from drying out. Spread 1 cup of the cheese mixture evenly over the pastry.
6. Layer two sheets of pastry over the cheese mixture, spraying each sheet with oil. Spread another cup of the cheese mixture evenly over the pastry. Repeat layering with two more layers of pastry and the remaining cheese mixture. Place the remaining three sheets of pastry on top of the cheese mixture, spraying each sheet with the cooking spray. Tuck the edges in.
7. Whisk the remaining egg lightly; brush over the top of the pie. Combine the seeds in a small bowl, sprinkle on the pie; bake for 40 minutes or until golden and cooked through.
8. Serve the pie with Greek yogurt and lemon wedges.

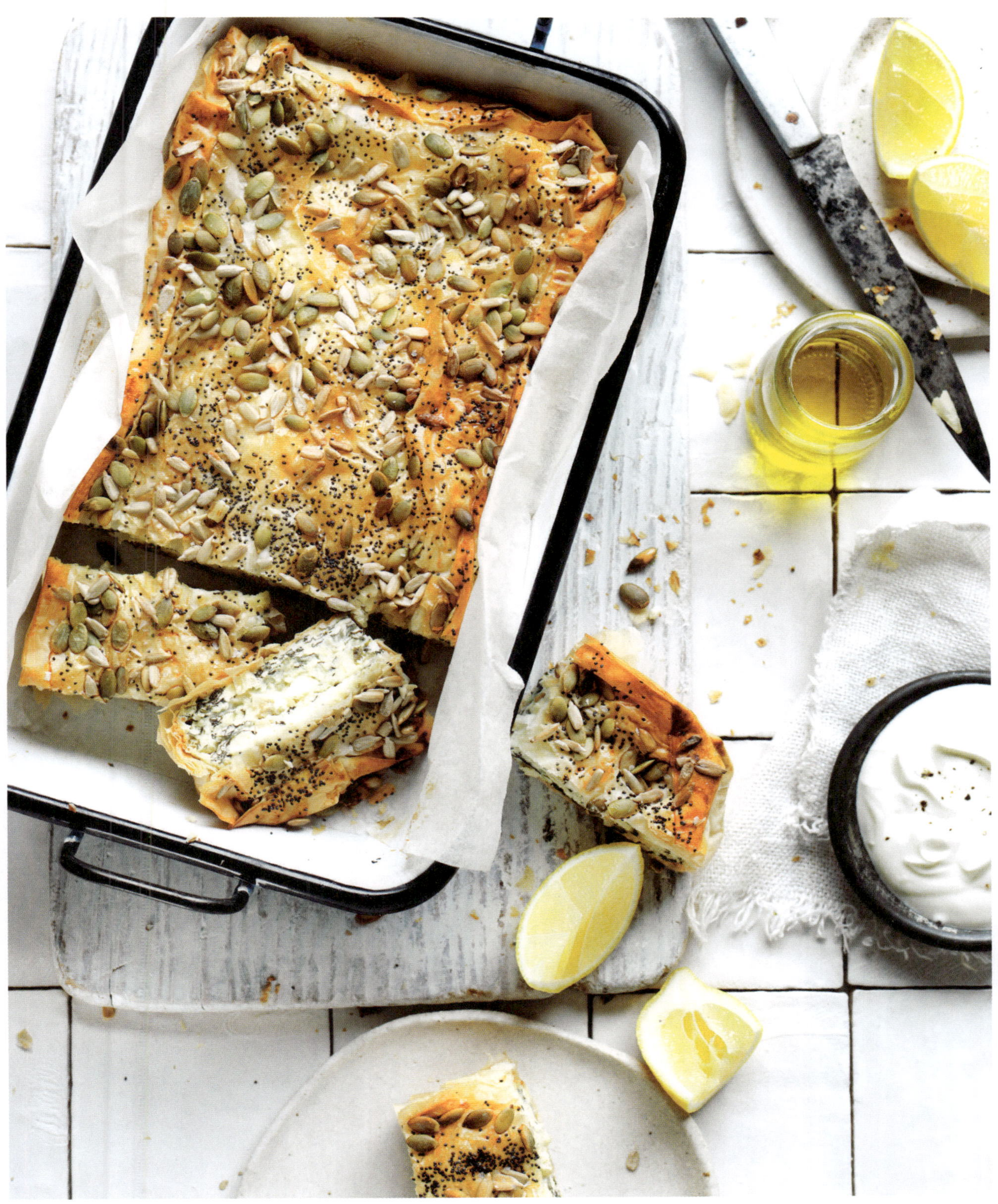

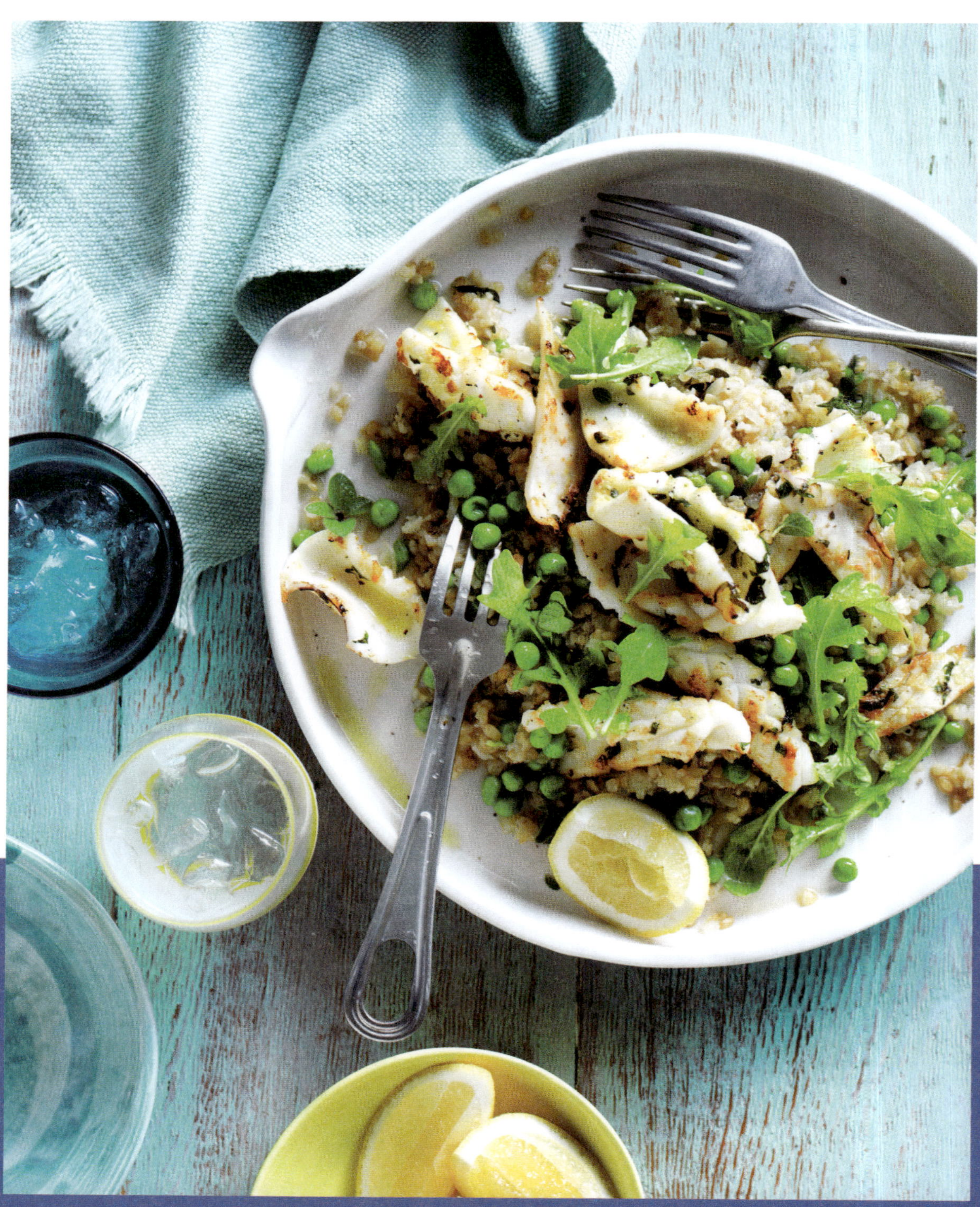

WEEKEND ENTERTAINING

Stunning fresh ingredients and classic Mediterranean flavors give these dishes the wow factor, adding finesse to a dinner party menu or a casual dinner with friends.

Gazpacho with feta cheese and shrimp

PESCATARIAN | PREP + COOK TIME **20 MINUTES** | SERVES **6**

The word gazpacho is derived from the Arabic for "soaked bread." It is a cold soup from southern Spain, made by blending raw vegetables. Gazpacho is traditionally served with accompaniments such as croutons, additional chopped vegetables, and chopped egg for diners to add as they wish. This luxurious version is instead topped with shrimp and feta.

2½lb (1.2kg) medium tomatoes, roughly chopped

2 red bell peppers, seeded and roughly chopped

1 medium cucumber, peeled, seeded, and roughly chopped

1 small onion, roughly chopped

3 garlic cloves, crushed

1 cup roughly chopped sourdough bread

1¼ cups olive oil, divided

½ cup red wine vinegar

1 cup water

salt and freshly ground black pepper

2lb (1kg) large cooked shrimp

4 slices sourdough bread, extra, crusts removed

½ cup feta cheese, crumbled

2 tbsp fresh oregano leaves

1. In the bowl of a food processor or blender, add the tomatoes, red peppers, cucumber, onion, garlic, bread, 1 cup of the olive oil, the vinegar, and the water. Pulse or blend on high until smooth. Season with salt and pepper to taste.
2. Peel and devein the shrimp, leaving the tails intact.
3. Tear the extra sourdough into coarse pieces. Heat 2 tbsp of the olive oil in a large skillet over medium-high heat. Cook the bread, stirring frequently, for 2 minutes or until the croutons are golden.
4. Ladle the soup into serving bowls; top with the croutons, feta cheese, shrimp, and oregano leaves. Drizzle the soup with the remaining oil.

TIP

Use the ripest tomatoes you can find to maximize the flavor of this classic Spanish soup.

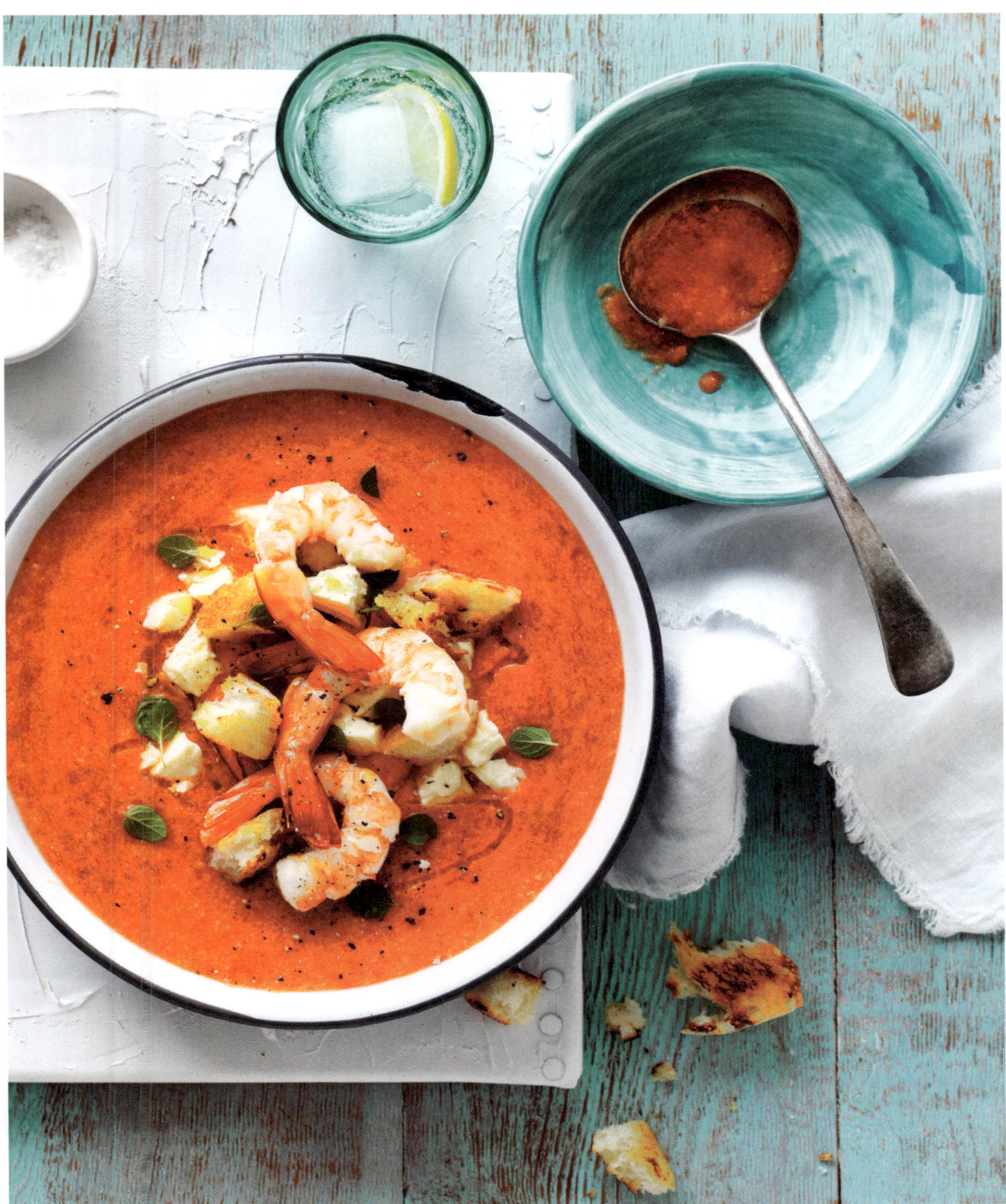

Chicken skewers with peach caprese salad

PREP + COOK TIME **25 MINUTES** | SERVES **4**

A traditional caprese salad, delicious in its simplicity, is comprised of layers of sliced fresh mozzarella, basil, and luscious sun-ripened tomatoes and traditionally served as an antipasto. This caprese is a little more substantial with the addition of grilled chicken skewers and peaches, which complement the richness of the buffalo mozzarella.

1lb (450g) boneless, skinless chicken breasts, cut into 1in (2.5cm) pieces

1½ tbsp olive oil (see tips)

salt and freshly ground black pepper

4 medium peaches

8oz (250g) buffalo mozzarella, torn into 1in (2.5cm) pieces (see tips)

2 medium tomatoes, sliced

1lb (450g) mixed heirloom cherry tomatoes, halved, quartered if large (see tips)

½ cup fresh small basil leaves

1 tbsp white wine vinegar

pistachio mint pesto

½ cup pistachios

1½ cups fresh mint leaves

1 cup fresh flat-leaf parsley leaves

1 garlic clove, crushed

2 tsp finely grated lemon rind

2 tsp lemon juice

½ cup extra virgin olive oil

TIPS

- You can use chile-infused olive oil for marinating the chicken, if you like.
- Buffalo mozzarella has a tangier flavor than cow's milk mozzarella, which may be used instead.
- You may swap regular cherry tomatoes for heirloom tomatoes, if preferred.

1. Make the pistachio mint pesto. In a food processor or blender, add all the ingredients and blend or pulse until smooth; season with salt and pepper to taste.
2. Cut the sides off the peaches in fat slices, cutting as close to the pit as possible. Discard the pits.
3. Combine the chicken and 1 tbsp of the olive oil in a medium bowl; season with salt and pepper. Thread onto four skewers.
4. Cook the chicken on a heated grill (barbecue) or ridged grill pan for 8 minutes. At that point, add the peaches to the grill or grill pan; cook for 2 minutes or until the chicken is cooked through and the peaches are golden and have grill marks.
5. Layer the grilled peaches with the mozzarella, tomatoes and basil; drizzle with the vinegar and remaining olive oil. Serve the salad topped with the chicken and pesto.

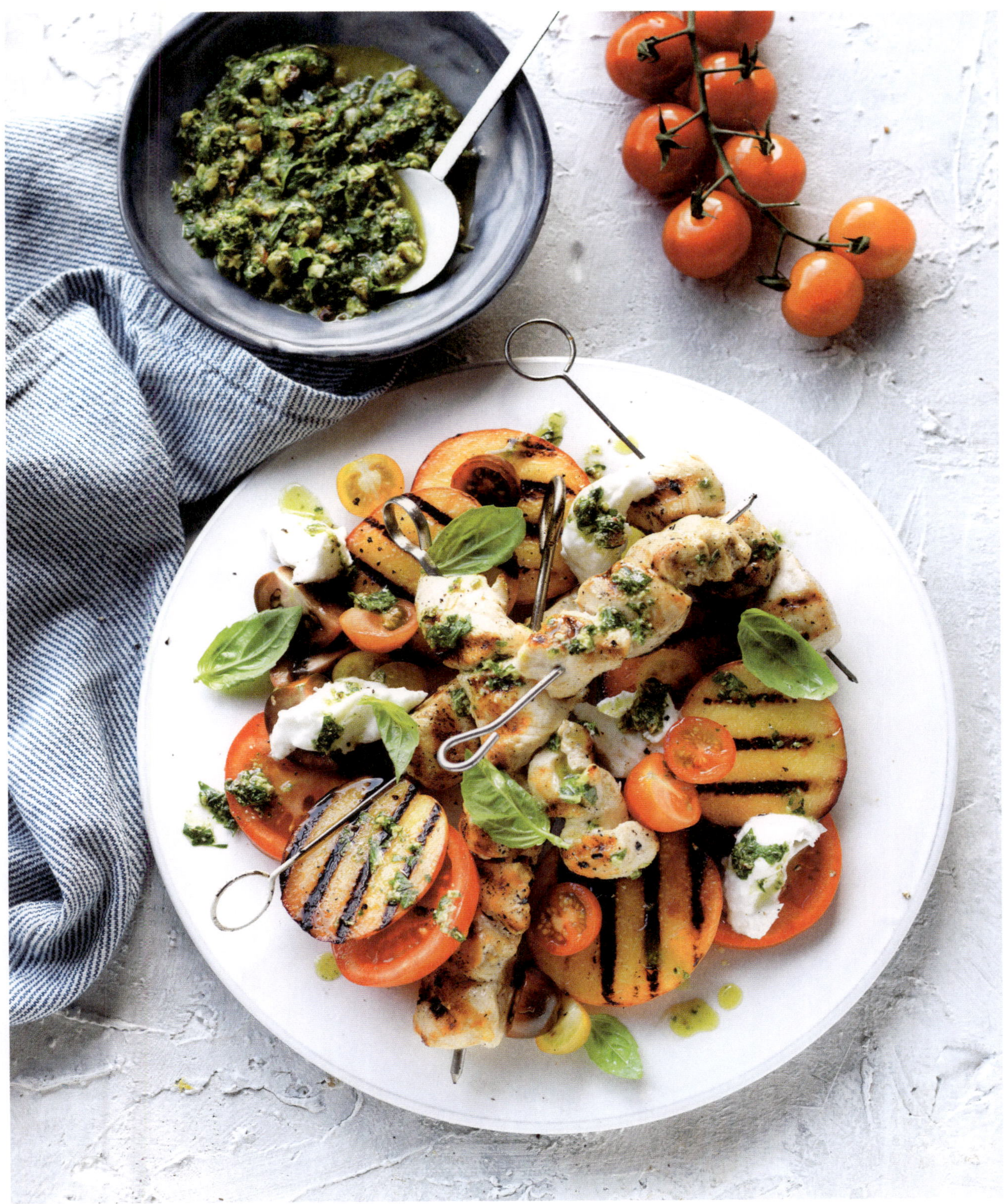

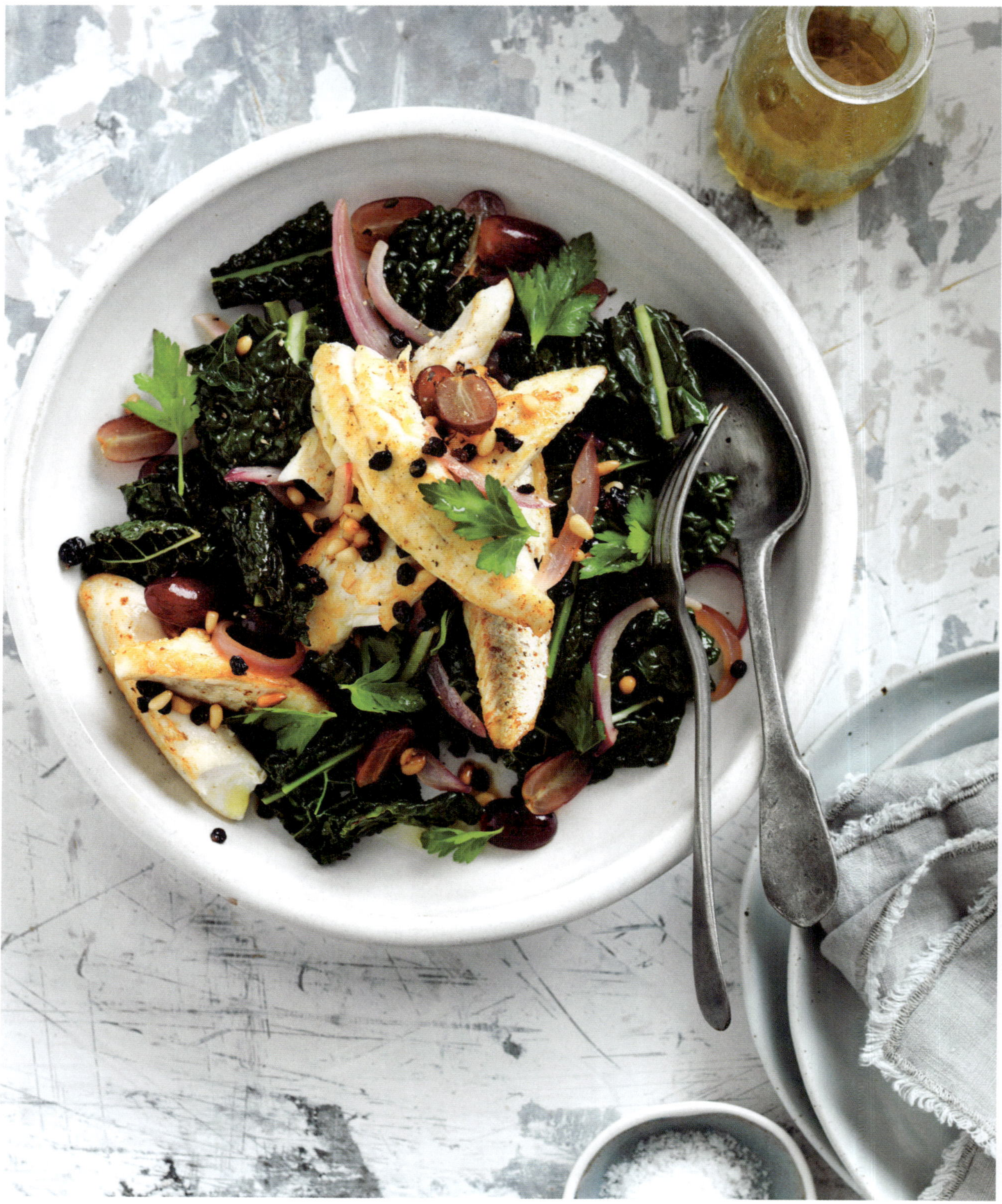

Fish with pine nuts, currants, and Tuscan kale

PESCATARIAN | PREP + COOK TIME **25 MINUTES** | SERVES **4**

This *agro dolce* (sweet and sour) Italian recipe uses dried currants and grapes for sweetness and vinegar for a sour note. Grapes contain powerful antioxidants known as polyphenols, which may slow or prevent many types of cancer. The resveratrol found in red wine—famous for heart health—is a type of polyphenol present in the skins of red grapes.

1/3 cup olive oil, divided
1 medium red onion, halved, sliced thinly
1 cup seedless red grapes, halved
2 tbsp dried currants
10oz (300g) Tuscan kale, trimmed, roughly chopped
1/4 cup red wine vinegar
1/3 cup pine nuts, toasted
salt and freshly ground black pepper
2lb (1kg) skinless, firm white fish fillets (see tip)
fresh Italian parsley sprigs, to garnish

1. Heat 1/4 cup of the oil in a large deep skillet over medium-high heat; cook onion for 4 minutes or until softened. Add grapes and dried currants; cook for 1 minute. Add kale and vinegar; cook, stirring, for 1 minute or until the kale just wilts. Add pine nuts. Season with salt and pepper. Set aside.
2. Heat remaining oil in the same skillet over medium-high heat; cook fish, in two batches, for 1 1/2 minutes on each side or until just cooked through. Season with salt and pepper.
3. Serve fish with kale mixture, sprinkled with parsley.

TIP

You can use any white-fleshed fish, such as bass, halibut, whiting, or john dory.

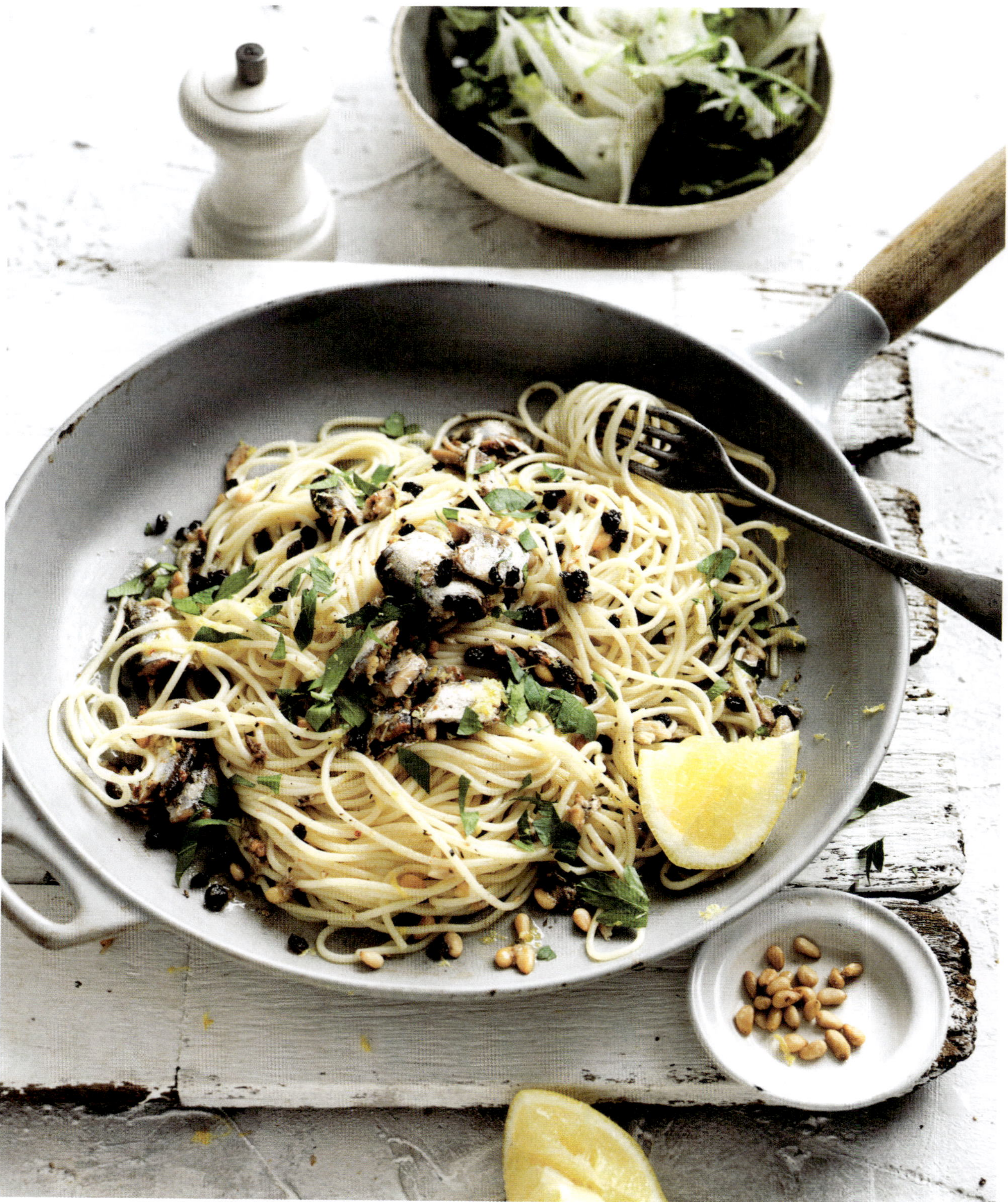

Chili sardine pasta with pine nuts and currants

PESCATARIAN | PREP + COOK TIME **20 MINUTES** | SERVES **4**

Dried fruits have long been an important component of the Mediterranean diet, eaten on their own or in traditional dishes. True currants are from the region of Corinth, and are small and black with an intense sweet flavor. Greece is still the primary producer of currants, with about 80 percent of total world production coming from that country.

16oz spaghetti (450g)

1/3 cup olive oil, divided

8oz (240g) canned sardines in lemon, chili, or garlic oil (see tips)

1/4 cup pine nuts, toasted

1/4 cup currants

2 tbsp lemon juice

salt and freshly ground black pepper

2 tsp finely grated lemon zest

1/2 cup fresh Italian parsley leaves, roughly chopped

4 cups arugula

1 fennel bulb, trimmed, thinly sliced (see tips)

lemon wedges, for serving

1. Cook the pasta in a large pot of boiling salted water until almost al dente; drain, reserving 1 cup of the cooking water.
2. Meanwhile, heat 1/4 cup of the olive oil in a large pan over medium heat. Add the sardines; cook, stirring occasionally, for 2 minutes or until heated through.
3. Add the pasta, pine nuts, currants, and lemon juice to the sardines. Heat pan over high heat. Add enough reserved water to moisten the pasta; cook, stirring, for 2 minutes. Season with salt and pepper to taste.
4. Combine the lemon zest and parsley in a small bowl; stir half through the pasta.
5. Place the arugula and fennel in a bowl to make a salad.
6. Divide the pasta among four bowls; sprinkle with the remaining lemon zest mixture and drizzle with the remaining olive oil. Serve with the arugula and fennel salad and lemon wedges.

TIPS

- Sardines in flavored oils are available in large supermarkets, gourmet shops, or specialty stores.
- Use a mandoline or V-slicer to slice the fennel very thinly.

Lamb, spinach, and feta cheese pie

PREP + COOK TIME **1 HOUR 20 MINUTES + STANDING** | SERVES **6**

The filling for this pie is quintessentially Greek with its flavorful tomato-based lamb sauce. This at-home take on a Greek classic uses premade pie crust for an easy weeknight meal. The decorative woven top makes it festive enough to serve to guests. It can be made ahead and refrigerated, then baked immediately before serving.

1/4 cup olive oil
2 medium onions, finely chopped
3 celery stalks, ribs trimmed and finely chopped
4 garlic cloves, crushed
2lb (1kg) ground lamb
1/2 cup dry red wine
1 1/2 cups vegetable stock
2 x 15oz (425g) can chopped tomatoes
1/3 cup tomato paste
1 tbsp chopped fresh oregano leaves
2 cinnamon sticks
5oz (150g) feta cheese, crumbled
3 cups spinach leaves, chopped
salt and freshly ground black pepper
14oz (400g) refrigerated pie crust (2 sheets), thawed slightly
1 egg
1 egg yolk
1 tsp sea salt flakes
1 tsp fennel seeds

1. Preheat oven to 425°F (220°C).
2. Heat the olive oil in a large pan over medium heat; cook the onion and celery, stirring, for 5 minutes or until lightly browned. Add the garlic; cook for 1 minute.
3. Increase heat to high, add the lamb; cook, stirring, until browned, breaking it up with the back of a wooden spoon. Add the wine; cook for 2 minutes. Add the stock, tomatoes, tomato paste, oregano, and cinnamon; cook for 15–20 minutes or until the liquid is evaporated and the sauce is thick. Cool.
4. Stir the feta cheese and spinach into the lamb mixture, season with salt and pepper to taste. Spoon the mixture into a 9in (23cm) round deep pie dish or 9 x 9in (23 x 23cm) heatproof casserole.
5. Roll out each of the round pie crusts on a floured surface. Using a sharp knife or pizza cutter, cut the pastry into 2in (5cm) wide strips. Starting in the center of the pie with the longest strips, weave strips over and under each other to create a lattice top. Let the edges overlap for a rustic effect. Brush the pastry with the combined beaten egg and egg yolk; sprinkle with salt and the fennel seeds.
6. Bake the pie for 25 minutes or until the pastry is a deep gold; cover the pastry with foil if it starts to brown too much. Let stand for 10 minutes before serving.

TIPS

- If minced lamb isn't available in your grocery's meat case, ask the butcher to grind some for you.
- You can replace the spinach with Swiss chard or kale; simply discard the tough center stalks first.

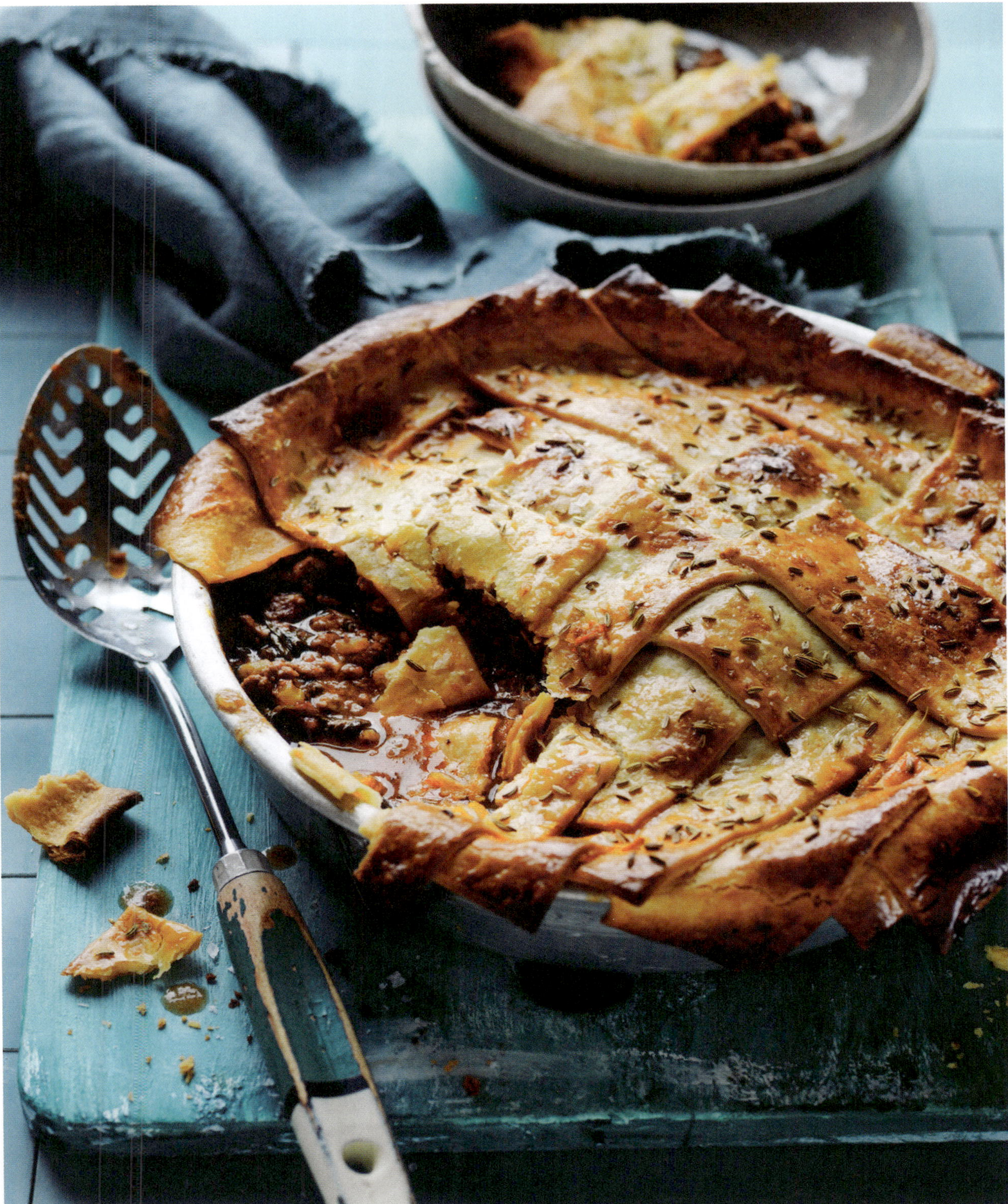

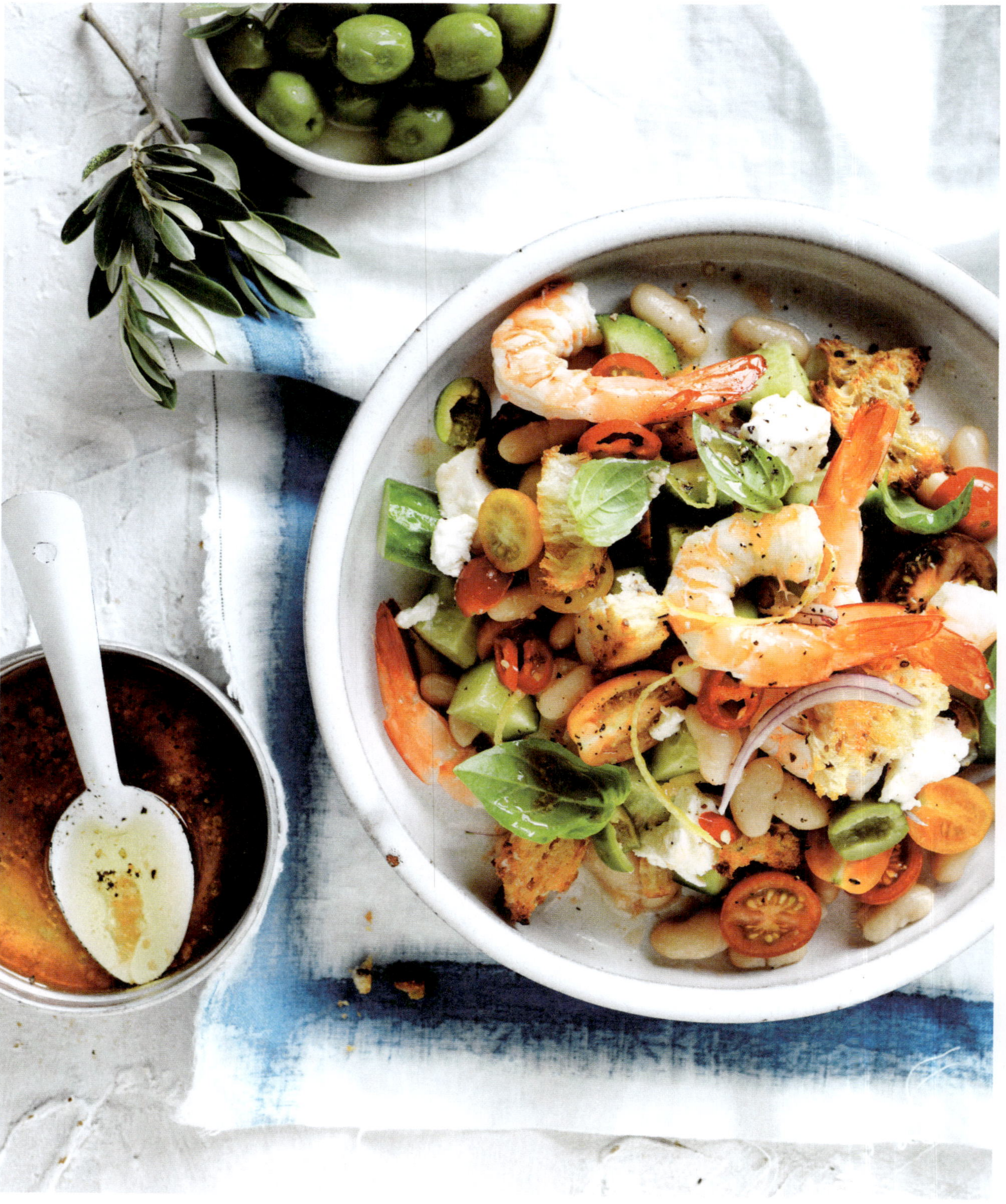

Spicy shrimp and white bean panzanella

PESCATARIAN | PREP + COOK TIME **20 MINUTES** | SERVES **4**

Before the advent of modern supermarket bread, every cuisine around the world had a recipe for using stale bread—panzanella is Italy's answer to this age-old problem. While starting off as a simple peasant dish born of necessity, panzanella has long been a dish favored for its simplicity, which allows the flavors of good-quality ingredients to shine through.

3–4 thick slices of whole grain sourdough bread, or any day-old bread
olive oil cooking spray
1 medium lemon
2lb (800g) cooked large shrimp
1 x 15oz (425g) can cannellini or Great Northern beans, drained and rinsed
10oz (250g) mixed cherry tomatoes, halved
1 medium cucumber, seeded and roughly chopped
1 small red onion, thinly sliced
1/2 cup pitted Sicilian olives, halved
1 fresh long red chile, thinly sliced
1 cup fresh basil leaves
4oz (120g) soft goat cheese, crumbled
1/4 cup olive oil
1/3 cup red wine vinegar
1 garlic clove, crushed
salt and freshly ground black pepper

1. Preheat oven to 425°F (220°C). Line a baking sheet with parchment paper.
2. Tear the bread coarsely into bite-sized pieces; place on the lined tray, spray with oil. Bake for 5 minutes or until golden and crisp.
3. Remove the zest from the lemon in long thin strips using a zester (see tips). Peel and devein the shrimp, leaving the tails intact.
4. Place the bread, lemon zest, shrimp, beans, tomatoes, cucumber, onion, olives, chile, basil, and half the goat cheese in a large bowl; toss gently to combine.
5. Combine the olive oil, vinegar, and garlic in a small bowl; season with salt and pepper to taste. Just before serving, spoon the dressing over the salad; top with the remaining cheese.

TIPS

- If you don't have a zester, you can finely grate the lemon rind instead.
- You could use marinated feta cheese instead of goat cheese.
- If you like, omit the shrimp and use a can of flaked drained tuna in olive oil instead.

Spanish-style fish with smoky eggplant

PESCATARIAN | PREP + COOK TIME **55 MINUTES + STANDING** | SERVES **4**

Red mullet is a fish particularly favored in Mediterranean cuisine for its delicate flavor and beautiful color. Eggplant is rich in anthocyanins, flavonoids that reduce blood pressure and lower risk of cardiovascular disease. It also possesses an abundance of nasunin an antioxidant, in its bright purple skin.

1 medium eggplant
1 red bell pepper
salt and freshly ground black pepper
1 tsp smoked paprika
2 tbsp olive oil, divided
2lb (900g) red mullet fillets, skin on (see tip)
1 x 15oz (425g) can cannellini or Great Northern beans, drained, rinsed
1/2 cup mayonnaise
1 garlic clove, crushed
1 tbsp lemon juice
1/4 cup fresh Italian parsley leaves
3 lemons

1 Preheat the oven to 400°F (200°C). Line a baking sheet with parchment paper.

2 Cut the eggplant in half lengthwise; score flesh at 1/2 in (1cm) intervals. Quarter the red bell pepper; discard seeds and membranes. Place the eggplant halves and pepper quarters, skin-side up, on the lined tray. Roast for 30 minutes or until the pepper's skin blisters and blackens and the eggplant is tender. Transfer to a heat-resistant bowl; cover for 5 minutes. Peel away the vegetable skins. Shred the eggplant coarsely; cut the pepper into thick slices. Season with salt and pepper to taste.

3 Meanwhile, combine the smoked paprika and 1 tbsp of the olive oil in a medium shallow bowl, add the fish; turn to coat. Heat a large nonstick skillet over high heat; cook the fish, in two batches, skin-side first, for 1½ minutes each side or until just cooked through. Transfer to a plate; let stand, covered loosely with foil.

4 Heat the remaining olive oil in the same pan over medium heat; cook the beans, stirring, until warmed through. Add the roasted eggplant and red pepper. Stir until just combined. Season with salt and pepper to taste. Set aside.

5 Combine the mayonnaise, garlic, and lemon juice in a small bowl to make aioli; season with salt and pepper to taste.

6 Meanwhile, cut lemon sides, which are seedless. Hold the fruit vertically. Place a knife at the top, 1/2 in (1cm) in to one side, and slice down, avoiding the core. Repeat around the fruit.

7 Put the bean, eggplant, and pepper mixture on each plate. Top with the fish and parsley. Serve with the aioli and lemon cheeks (see photo).

TIP

You may use bream, Mediterranean sea bass (loup de mer), or other white fish fillets instead of red mullet, if you like.

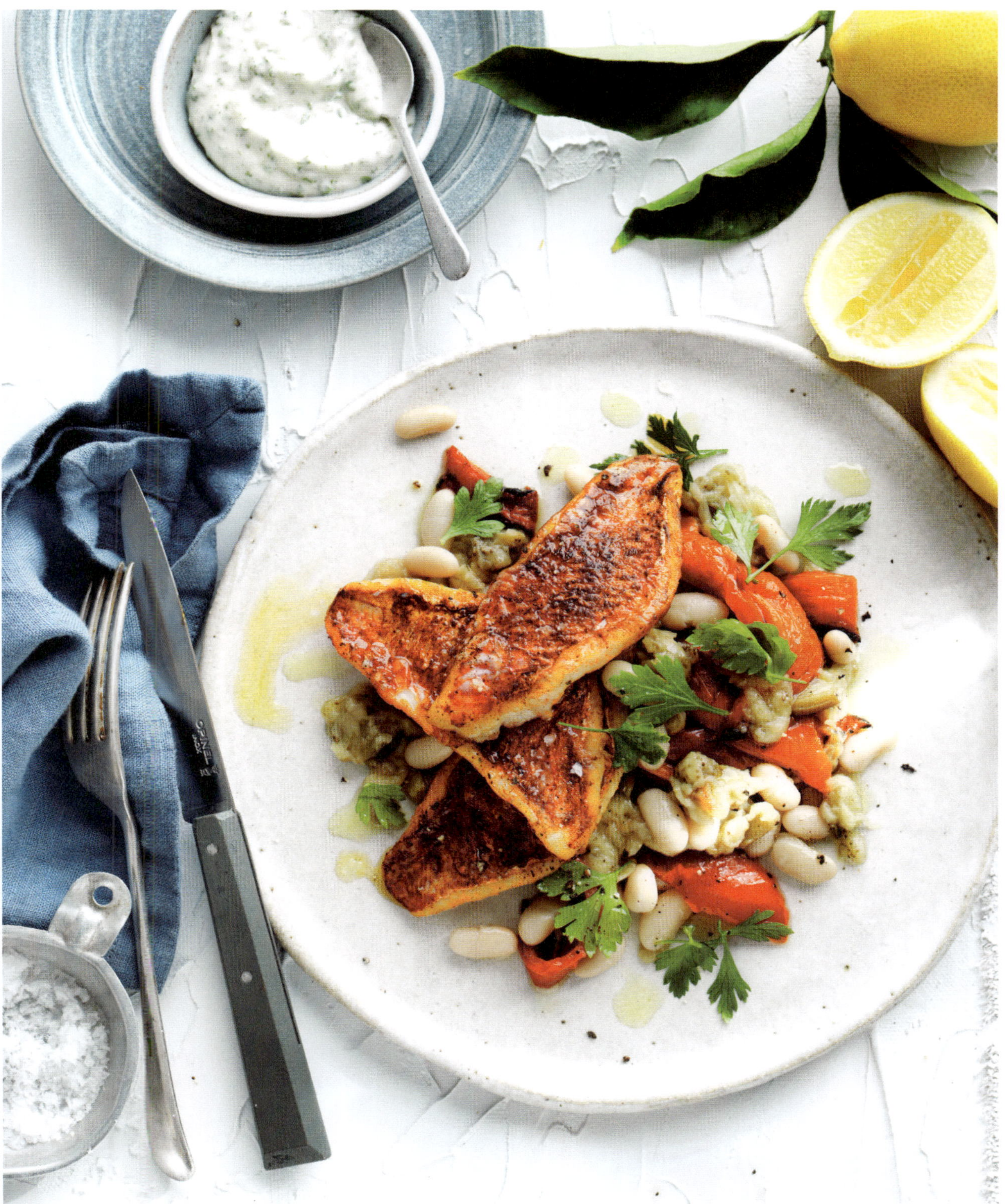
OPINEL

Lamb with spinach pesto dressing

PREP + COOK TIME **35 MINUTES** | SERVES **4**

Lamb contains many nutrients, such as iron, zinc, selenium, and vitamin B12, and is also an excellent source of protein. If your supermarket doesn't stock it, try your local farmer's market, butcher, or gourmet grocery. Whenever possible, look for locally produced or grass-fed lamb, because it packs an extra nutritional punch while benefiting local producers.

1½lb (680g) boneless lamb loin
1 garlic clove, crushed
salt and freshly ground black pepper
1 tbsp olive oil
½ small red onion, cut into thin wedges
3 medium heirloom tomatoes, quartered
1 cup arugula
½ cup marinated soft goat cheese, reserve 2 tbsp of the marinating oil (see tips)

spinach pesto dressing

½ cup spinach pesto (see tips)
¼ cup olive oil

1. Combine the lamb, garlic, and olive oil in a medium bowl; season with salt and pepper.
2. Cook the onion on a heated grill (barbecue) or ridged grill pan until browned and just tender; season with salt and pepper to taste. Cover loosely with foil to keep warm.
3. Cook the lamb on the heated grill (barbecue) or ridged grill pan, turning occasionally, for 10 minutes for medium or until cooked as desired. Let stand, covered loosely with foil, for 5 minutes. Slice thickly.
4. Meanwhile, to make the spinach pesto dressing, place the ingredients in a small screw-top jar; shake well. Season with salt and pepper to taste.
5. Place the onion, tomato, arugula, and reserved marinating oil in a large bowl; toss gently to combine. Season with salt and pepper to taste.
6. Add the lamb to the salad; toss to combine. Arrange salad on a platter. Top with the crumbled cheese; drizzle with the dressing.

TIPS

- The oil from the marinated goat cheese adds extra depth of flavor to this dish. The cheese we used was marinated in a mixture of olive oil, garlic, thyme, and chili.
- You can use any pesto, including your favorite store-bought brand.

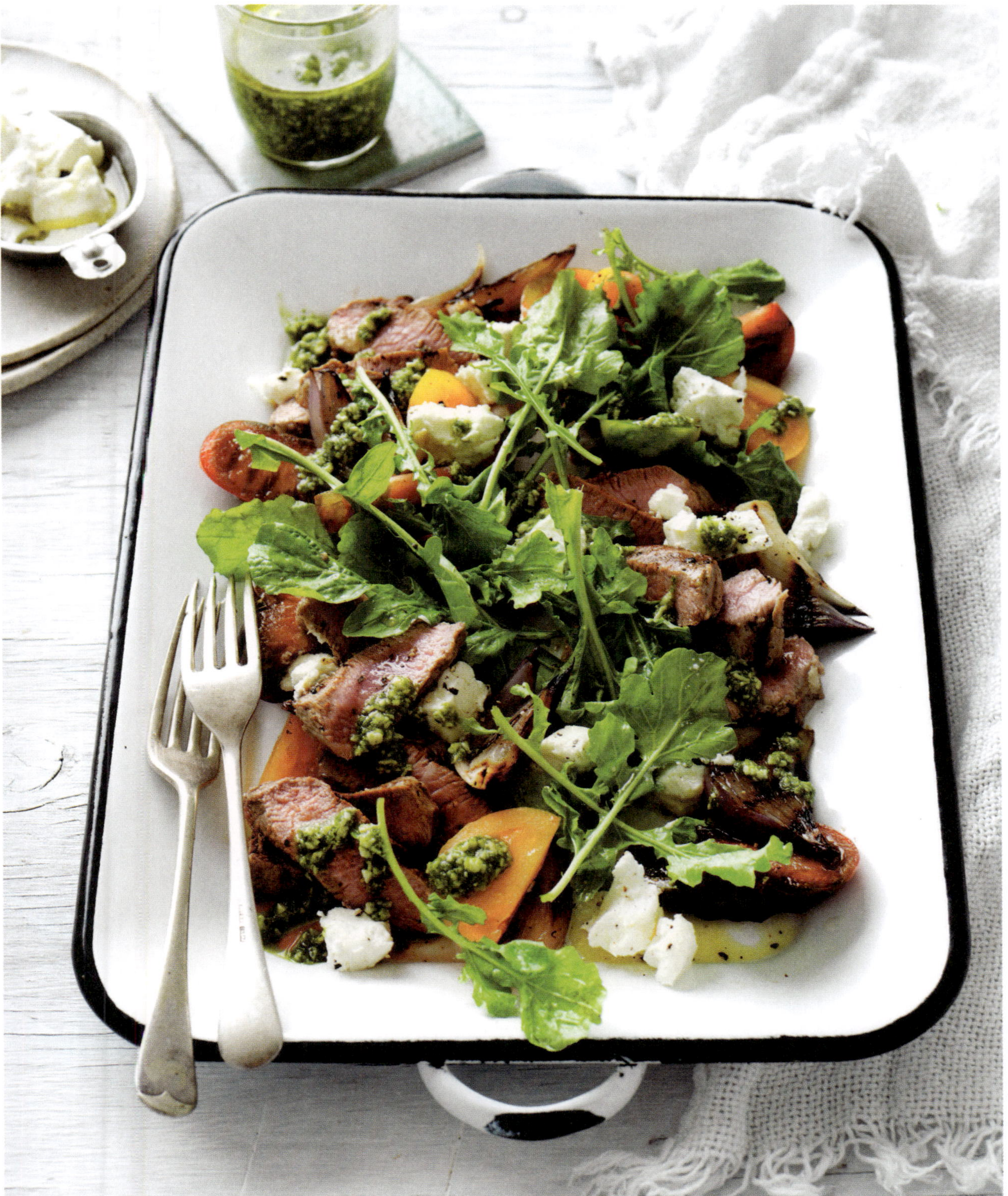

Pan-fried fish with tomato and olive salsa

PESCATARIAN | PREP + COOK TIME **50 MINUTES** | SERVES **6**

This delicious seafood dish uses the Mediterranean staples of tomatoes and olives in a robust salsa. Use any firm white fish to serve as the foundation of the dish. With excellent olive oil and roasted potatoes, you'll have a delicious and nutrition-packed meal. Omega-3 fatty acids, which are abundant in seafood, help protect against heart disease and strokes.

2lb (900g) fingerling potatoes, halved lengthwise
2 tbsp red wine vinegar
1/4 cup olive oil, divided
1lb (450g) green beans, trimmed
1/2 cup all-purpose flour
salt and freshly ground black pepper
2lb (960g) white fish fillets, skin on
lemon wedges, to serve

tomato and olive salsa
1/3 cup olive oil, divided
2 garlic cloves, crushed
1lb (450g) grape tomatoes, halved
5oz (150g) pitted Kalamata olives, halved
1/2 small red onion, finely chopped
1/2 cup fresh Italian parsley leaves
2 tbsp lemon juice

1. Make the tomato and olive salsa. Heat 1 tbsp of the olive oil in a medium saucepan over medium heat; cook the garlic, stirring, until fragrant. Stir in the tomatoes and olives; cook until heated through. Remove from heat; stir in the onion, parsley, remaining olive oil, and lemon juice. Season with salt and pepper to taste. Set aside.

2. Place the potatoes in a large saucepan, cover with cold water; bring to a boil. Boil for 8 minutes or until tender; drain. Transfer to a large bowl; drizzle with the vinegar and 1 tbsp of the oil. Cover to keep warm.

3. Meanwhile, cook the green beans in a saucepan of boiling water for 3 minutes or until tender; drain. Plunge into a bowl of iced water; drain. Add to the potatoes in the bowl; toss gently to combine.

4. Season the flour with salt and pepper; coat the fish in the seasoned flour, shake off excess. Heat the remaining olive oil in a large frying pan over medium heat; cook fish, skin-side down, in batches, for 4 1/2 minutes or until skin crisps. Turn, cook for 1 more minute or until the fish is just cooked through.

5. Divide the potatoes and beans among the plates; top with the fish and salsa. Serve with lemon wedges.

TIP

The salsa can be partially prepared up to a day ahead; add the parsley, remaining oil, and lemon juice just before you cook the fish.

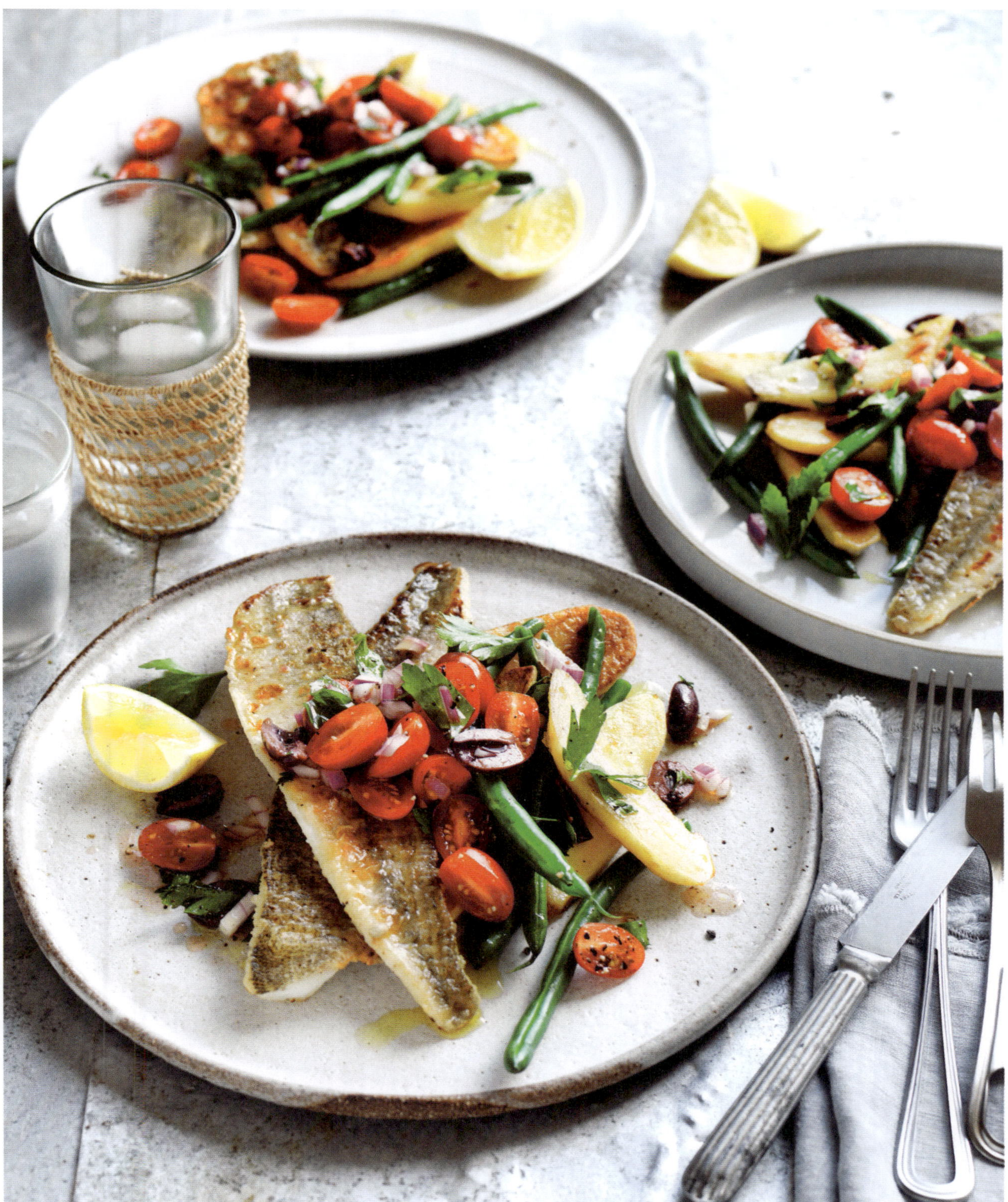

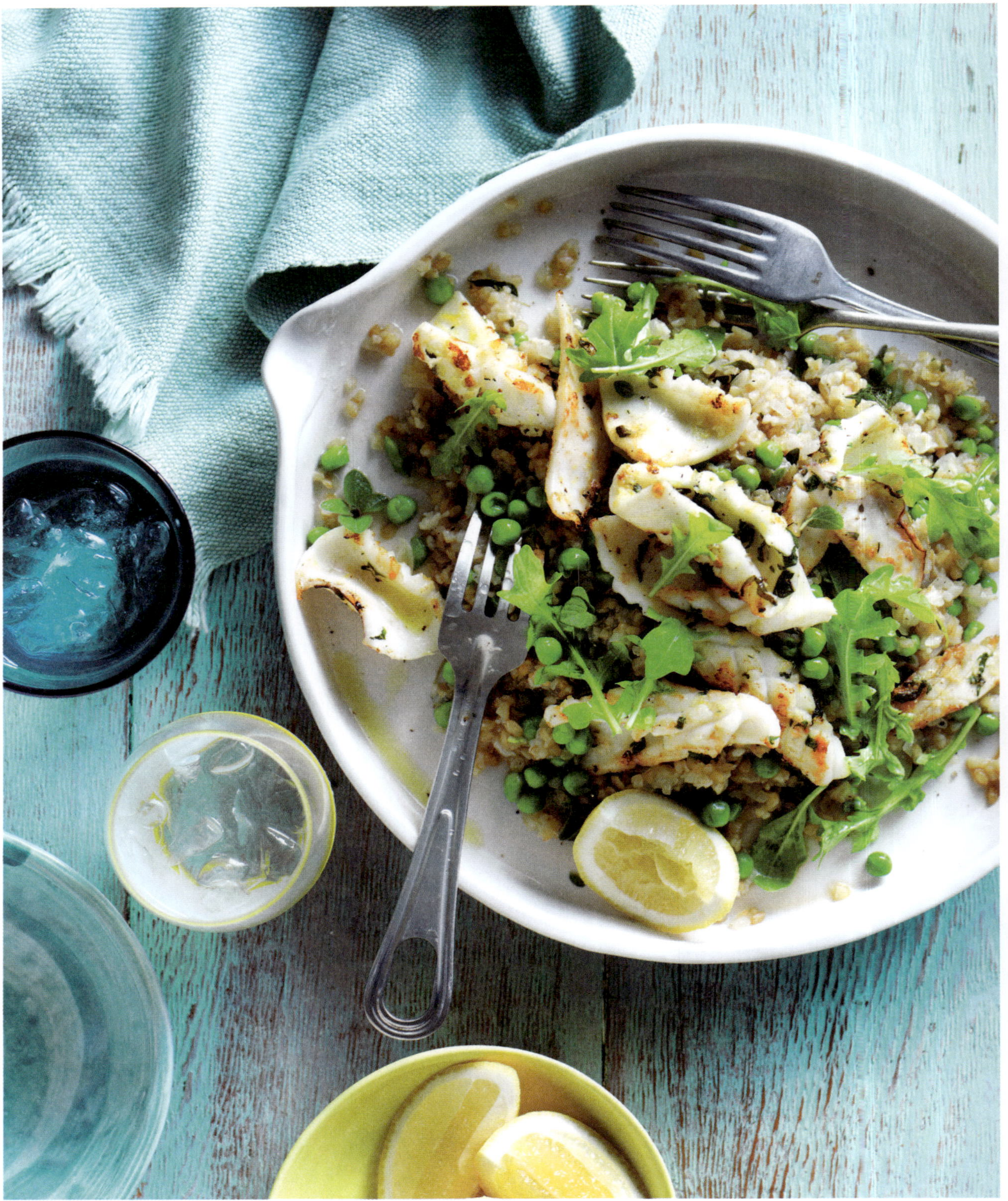

Grilled calamari with lemon cracked wheat risotto

PESCATARIAN | PREP + COOK TIME **45 MINUTES** | SERVES **2**

Bulgur is used extensively in Middle Eastern cuisine, but is also enjoyed throughout the Mediterranean region. Eaten as you would rice or couscous, bulgur has a coarse texture and nutty flavor, and can be used in soups, stews, and salads. It's low in fat, high in minerals and iron, and serves as a good source of plant-based protein.

10oz (300g) frozen or fresh calamari, cleaned (see tips)
3 garlic cloves, crushed
2 tsp chopped fresh oregano leaves
1 tsp finely grated lemon zest
2 tbsp olive oil, divided
1/2 cup onion, finely chopped
2 tsp fresh lemon thyme leaves
1/2 cup coarse bulgur
1 cup frozen peas
1 tbsp lemon juice
2 tsp fresh oregano leaves, extra

1. Using a sharp knife, score the inside surface of the calamari hood in a criss-cross pattern at 1/2in (1cm) intervals. Cut into 1 1/2in (4cm) strips. Place in a bowl with any additional calamari pieces, 1 garlic clove, the chopped oregano, lemon zest, and 1 tbsp of the olive oil; stir to combine.
2. Heat the remaining olive oil in a medium nonstick skillet over medium heat; cook the onion, remaining garlic, and thyme, stirring, for 5 minutes or until the onion is softened.
3. Add the bulgur and 2 cups of water; cook, stirring occasionally, for 15 minutes or until the bulgur is tender. Add the peas and lemon juice; cook, stirring, for 2 minutes or until heated through. Season with salt and pepper.
4. Meanwhile, cook the calamari on a heated grill (barbecue) or ridged grill pan for 2 minutes, or until just cooked through, turning halfway through the cooking time. Season with salt and pepper.
5. Serve the calamari with the bulgur mixture; sprinkle with the extra oregano.

TIPS

- For frozen calamari, thaw under running water before use. If you want to clean your own calamari, you will need a 2lb (900g) whole calamari.
- You could also try this recipe with thin strips of chicken or pork.

Fennel

Fennel is a flowering plant species in the carrot family. Grown for its edible bulbs, shoots, leaves, and seeds, it is used extensively in Mediterranean cooking. Aromatic and flavorful, it's also a rich source of fiber, protein, minerals, and B vitamins.

Maple-roasted fennel

VEGAN | PREP + COOK TIME **35 MINUTES** | SERVES **4**

Preheat the oven to 400°F (200°C). Reserve the green fennel fronds from 2 large fennel bulbs. Cut the fennel bulbs in half. Line a baking sheet with parchment paper. In a bowl, add 8 fresh thyme sprigs and 2 tbsp each of pure maple syrup and olive oil. Add the fennel halves; toss to combine. Turn the fennel cut-side down on the baking sheet. Season with salt and pepper. Roast for 25 minutes or until tender and browned. Serve the fennel drizzled with balsamic vinegar, topped with the chopped reserved fronds and 1/4 cup of roasted sliced almonds.

Shaved fennel slaw

VEGAN | PREP TIME **15 MINUTES** | SERVES **4**

Place 3 cups shredded green cabbage in a large bowl with 1 thinly shaved fennel bulb, 1 thinly sliced seeded green chile, and 1 cup each of fresh cilantro and fresh mint leaves; toss gently to combine. Combine 1/4 cup each of lemon juice and olive oil in a small bowl; season with salt and pepper to taste. Drizzle the dressing over the slaw; toss gently to combine.

Pickled fennel bruschetta

VEGETARIAN | PREP + COOK TIME **15 MINUTES + STANDING**
SERVES **4**

Place 1 medium thinly sliced fennel bulb in a medium bowl with 1 crushed garlic clove, 1/3 cup white balsamic vinegar, 2 tsp of sugar, and 6 thinly sliced red radishes; toss to combine. Let stand for 30 minutes. Drain. Spread 6oz (180g) drained feta cheese on 4 slices of chargrilled sourdough bread; top with the pickled fennel.

Grapefruit and fennel salad

VEGAN | PREP TIME **15 MINUTES** | SERVES **4**

Cut 1 pink grapefruit into segments. Place the grapefruit in a medium bowl with 1 thinly shaved fennel bulb and 1/4 cup of squashed Sicilian olives; toss gently to combine. Whisk 1/4 cup of grapefruit juice, 1 crushed garlic clove, 1 1/2 tbsp of sherry vinegar, and 2 tbsp of olive oil in a small bowl. Serve the salad drizzled with the dressing.

CLOCKWISE from top left

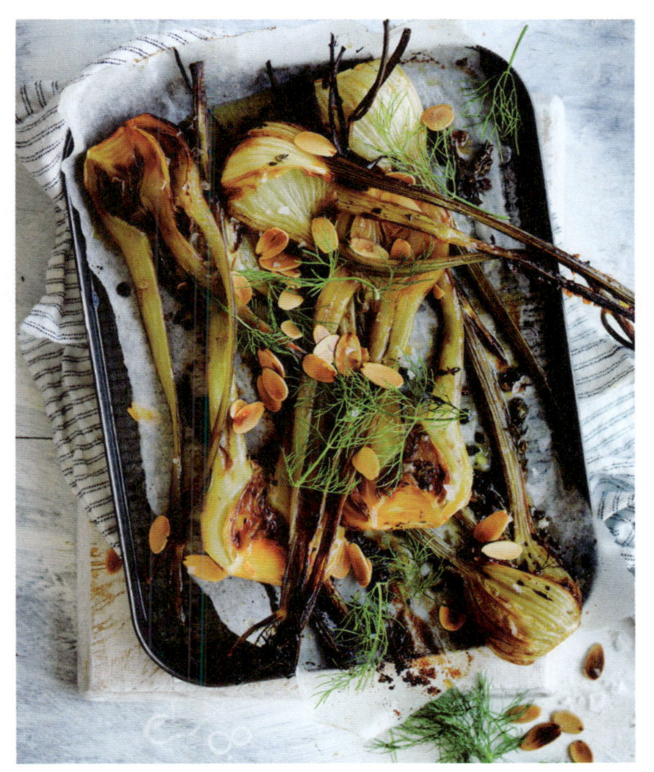

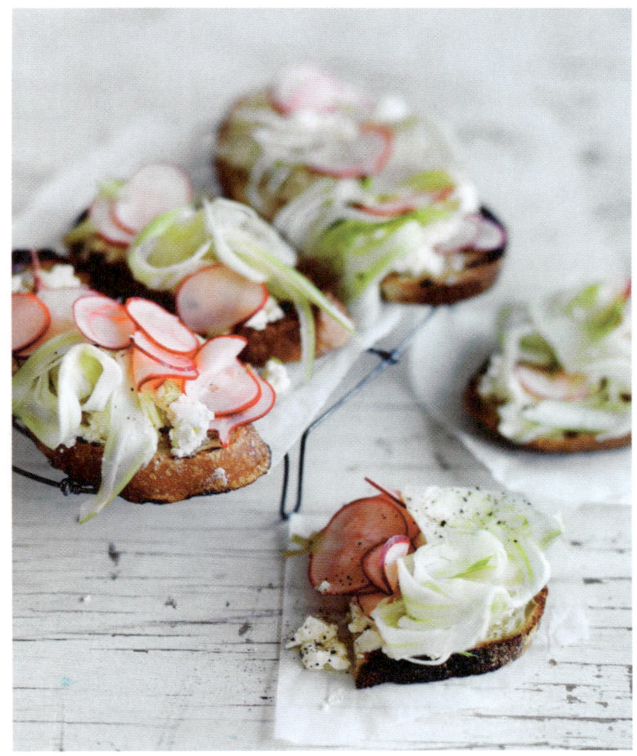

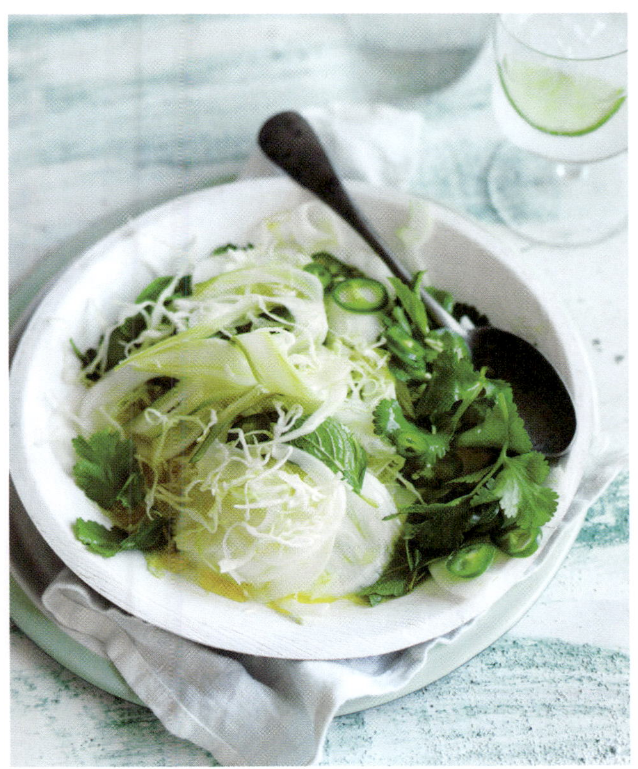

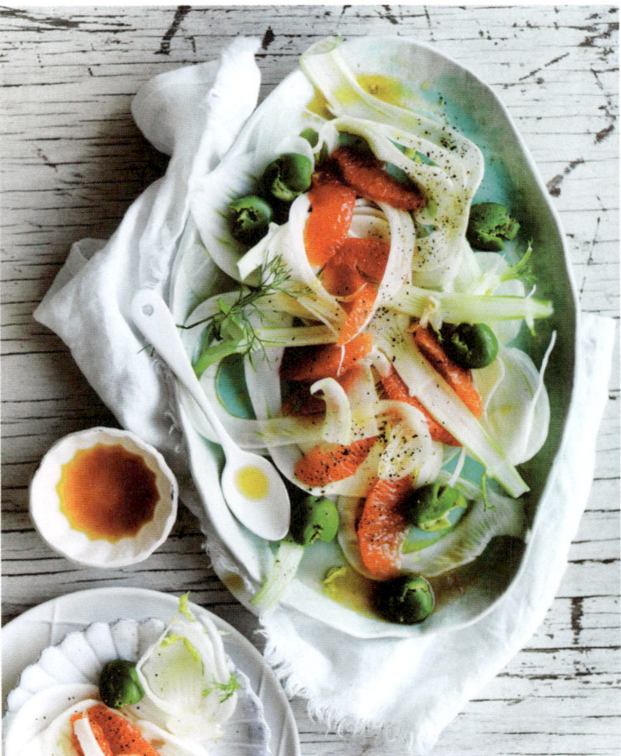

Lamb kefta with zucchini baba ganoush

PREP + COOK TIME **1 HOUR 15 MINUTES + REFRIGERATION** | SERVES **4**

Baba ganoush is traditionally a dish consisting of a mixture of smoky eggplant, tahini, olive oil, and various spices. This version replaces the eggplant with roasted zucchini for a lighter twist on the classic. Tahini is a paste made from toasted hulled sesame seeds and is available from most major supermarkets and Middle Eastern food stores.

1½lb (600g) boneless leg of lamb, coarsely ground (see tip)

1 egg

2 tsp ground cumin

1 garlic clove, crushed

¾ cup finely chopped fresh mint leaves, divided

salt and freshly ground black pepper

1 medium lemon, including zest and 1½ tbsp juice

1 cup pearl barley

1½ cups frozen peas

⅓ cup olive oil

mint leaves, extra, to garnish

zucchini baba ganoush

2 medium zucchini, untrimmed

1½ tbsp olive oil

1 tbsp tahini

½ tsp ground cumin

1 small garlic clove, crushed

TIP

You can ask your butcher to grind the lamb for you. For step 1, chilling the food processor bowl and blade in the freezer for 15 minutes before processing the kofta mixture ensures the mixture is nicely chopped and not mushy.

1. In the bowl of a food processor, add the lamb, egg, cumin, and garlic; pulse until finely chopped. Place in a large bowl with ¼ cup of chopped mint. Season with salt and pepper and knead for 2 minutes or until well combined. Divide the mixture into 8 portions. Shape the portions into keftas. Press onto skewers. Refrigerate for 1 hour.

2. Meanwhile, finely grate the zest from a lemon. Squeeze the juice; reserve 1½ tbsp of juice for the baba ganoush.

3. To make the zucchini baba ganoush, preheat oven to 425°F (220°C). Bake the whole zucchinis on a baking sheet for 40 minutes or until very soft and slightly blackened. In the bowl of a food processor, add the zucchini, the olive oil, tahini, cumin, garlic, and reserved lemon juice; pulse until smooth. Season with salt and pepper to taste. Set aside.

4. Place the pearl barley and 3 cups water in a medium saucepan, bring to a boil. Reduce heat to low; cook, covered, for 35 minutes or until tender. Drain. Cook the peas in a saucepan of boiling water for 2 minutes or until tender; drain.

5. In a large bowl, place the pearl barley, peas, lemon zest, remaining chopped mint, and 2 tbsp of olive oil; toss gently to combine. Season with salt and pepper to taste.

6. Brush the kefta with the remaining olive oil; cook on a heated grill (barbecue) or ridged grill plate over medium-high heat, turning, for 10 minutes or until cooked as desired.

7. Serve the kefta with the baba ganoush and pearl barley salad, sprinkled with mint.

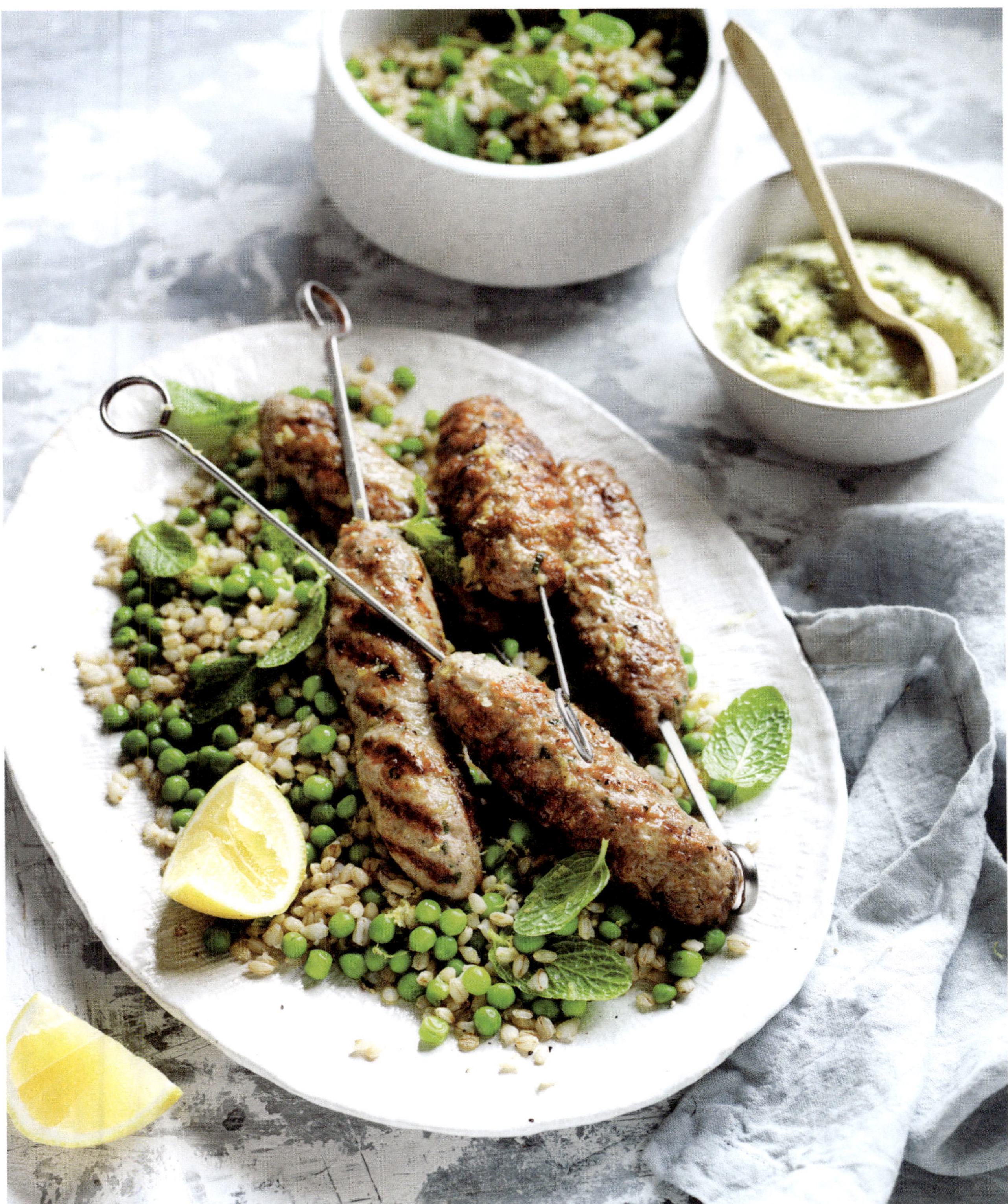

Roasted fish with celery root and fennel salad

PESCATARIAN | PREP + COOK TIME **1 HOUR + REFRIGERATION AND STANDING** | SERVES **8**

Roasting a whole fish may seem intimidating, but there really is nothing to it, and it makes quite an impression when plated and served. Juniper berries are not true berries, but are seeds produced by the various species of juniper trees. Used as a spice in European cuisine, they also give gin its distinctive flavor. They are the only spice to be derived from conifers.

8 whole small white fish (about 5½ lb [2.6kg]), cleaned (see tips)

salt and freshly ground black pepper

8 thyme sprigs, trimmed

2 garlic cloves, thinly sliced

1 tbsp dried juniper berries

¼ cup olive oil, divided

1 tbsp finely grated lemon zest or strips

4 lemons

celery root and fennel salad

1 medium celery root, peeled, cut into fine matchsticks (see tips)

2 fennel bulbs, trimmed, thinly sliced (see tips), fronds reserved

⅓ cup fresh Italian parsley leaves

⅓ cup lemon juice

¼ cup olive oil

1. Wash the fish inside and out, pat dry with paper towel. Season inside and out with salt and pepper. Score the fish three times on both sides, through the thickest part. Place on a baking sheet. Place a thyme sprig, some reserved fennel fronds, and a slice of garlic into each cut. Using a mortar and pestle, grind the juniper berries into a coarse powder. Coat the fish all over with 2 tbsp of the olive oil, the lemon zest, and the ground juniper berries. Refrigerate for 1 hour.
2. Meanwhile, to make the celery root and fennel salad, combine the ingredients in a large bowl; season with salt and pepper to taste.
3. Preheat oven to 350°F (180°C). Line a large baking sheet with parchment paper.
4. Brush the fish with the remaining olive oil; place on the lined baking sheet. Roast the fish for 18 minutes or until cooked through. Let stand, covered loosely with foil, for 5 minutes.
5. Meanwhile, cut lemon sides, which are nice to use because they're seedless. Hold the fruit vertically. Place a knife at the top ½in (1cm) in to one side, and slice down, avoiding the core. Repeat around the fruit.
6. Serve the fish with the salad and lemon sides.

TIPS

- If 8 small fish are not available, you can substitute 4 larger fish (or 2 quite large). Ask at the seafood counter to find out what's local and in season.
- Use a mandoline or V-slicer to quickly and easily cut the celery root into fine matchsticks and the fennel into thin slices.

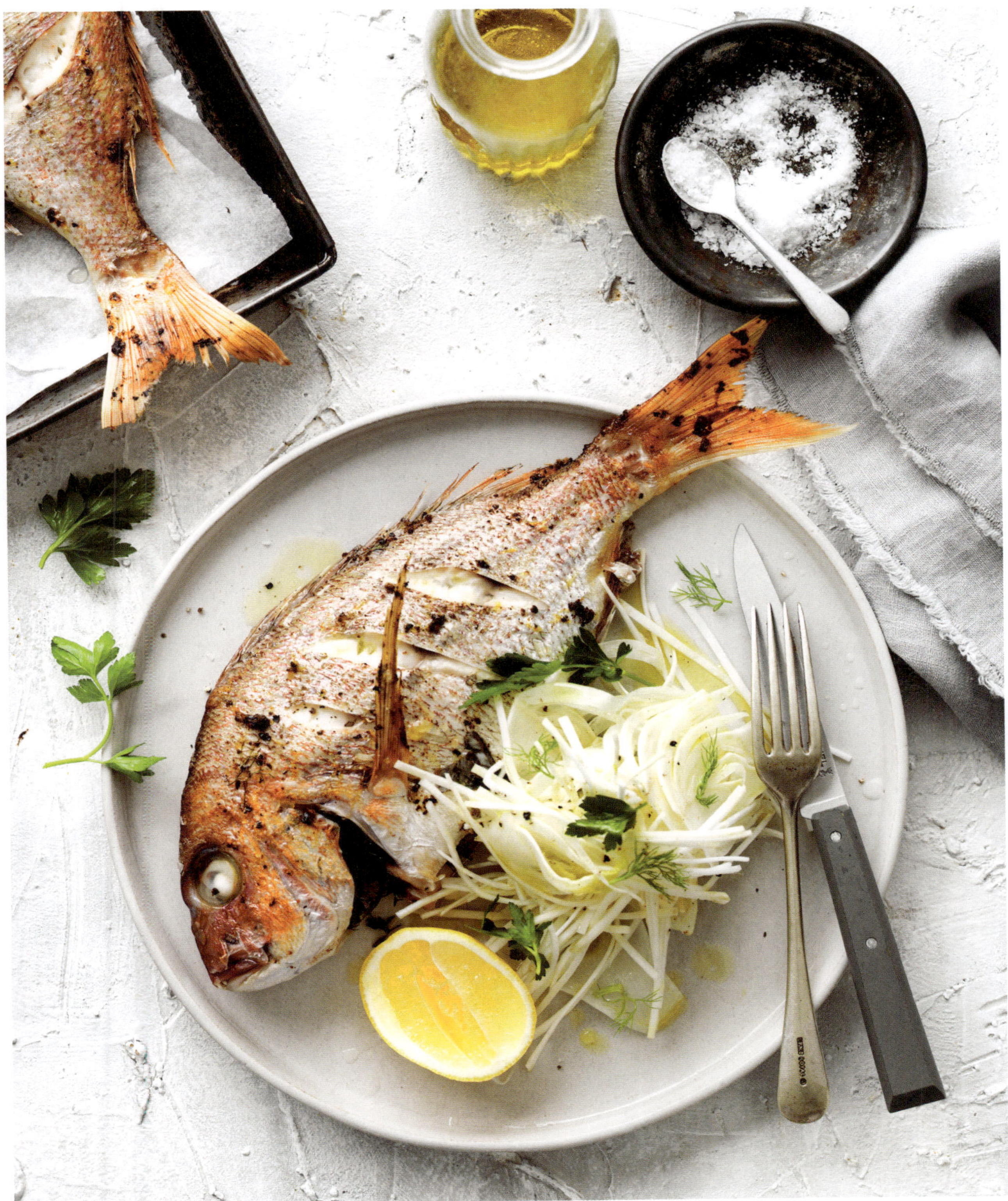

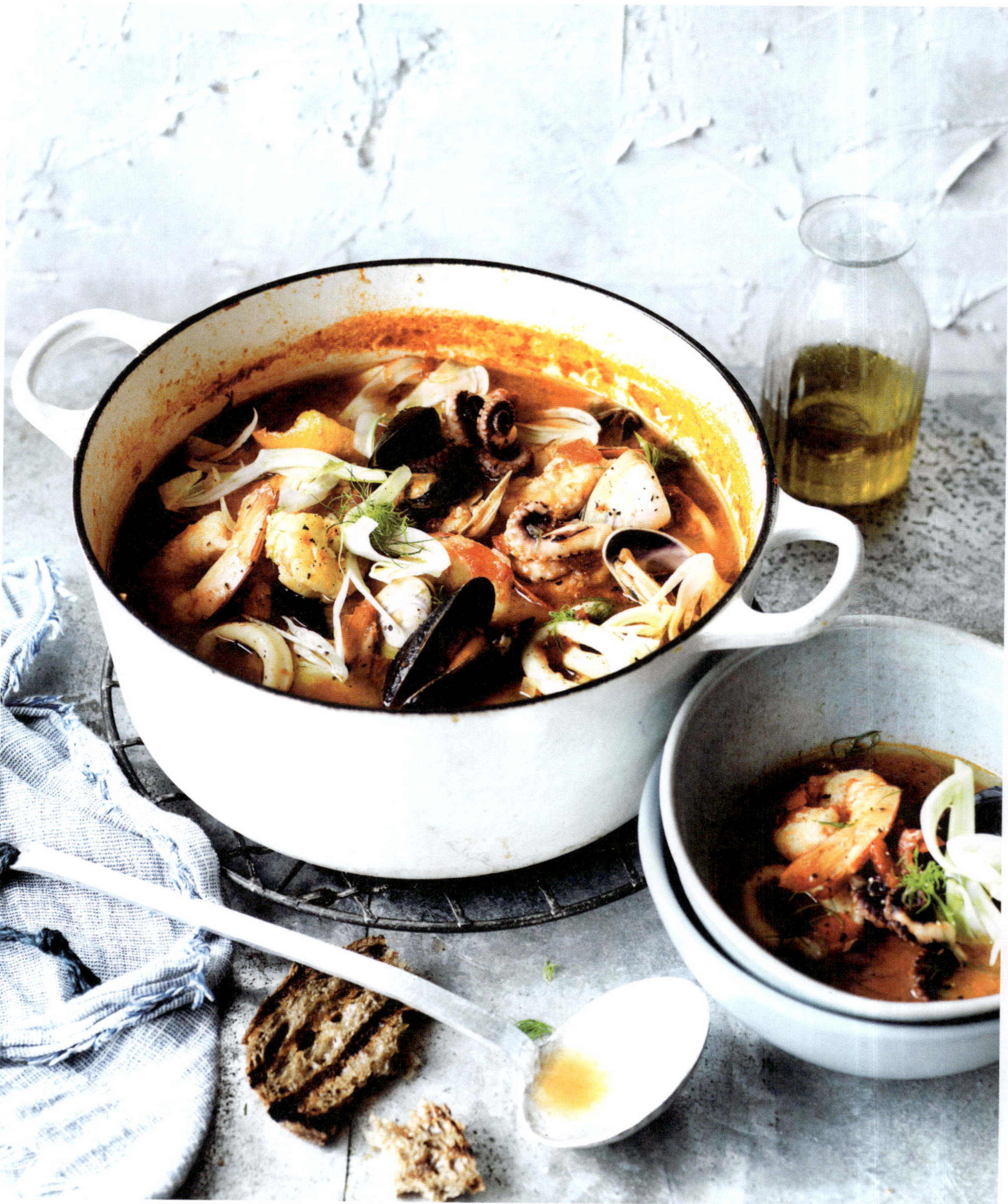

Seafood and saffron stew

PESCATARIAN | PREP + COOK TIME **1 HOUR** | SERVES **4**

This rich seafood stew combines mussels, clams, calamari, octopus, and shrimp to make a rich tomato seafood stew that includes everything from the day's catch. Variations exist all over the Mediterranean and have even made it to the new world. The saffron and orange in this hearty meal give you a flavor of southern Spain.

1lb (450g) frozen or fresh cleaned calamari
1lb (450g) fresh mussels, cleaned (see tips)
1 tbsp olive oil
1 large onion, finely chopped
2 garlic cloves, crushed
3 wide strips orange rind (see tips)
1 fresh long red chile, finely chopped
pinch of saffron threads
1/3 cup dry white wine
2 x 15oz (425g) cans diced tomatoes
4 cups fish stock
2lb (1 kg) uncooked large shrimp, peeled, deveined, with tails intact
1/2 lb (200g) clams, scrubbed
1/2 lb (200g) fresh or frozen octopus pieces
1 fennel bulb
2 tbsp lemon juice

1. Using a sharp knife, slice the calamari hoods crosswise into 1/2 in (1cm) rings. Scrub the mussels; remove beards. Discard any mussels with cracked or broken shells.
2. Heat the olive oil in a large stockpot; cook the onion, stirring, until soft. Add the garlic; cook, stirring, for 1 minute.
3. Add the orange rind, chile, saffron, and wine to the onion mixture; cook, stirring, for 2 minutes. Add the tomatoes; cook for 10 minutes or until the mixture thickens slightly. Add the stock; cook for 20 minutes or until the liquid is reduced by about a quarter.
4. Add the calamari, prawns, cleaned mussels, clams, and octopus to the pot. Cook, covered, stirring occasionally, for 5 minutes or until the seafood is just cooked.
5. Meanwhile, trim the fennel; reserve fronds. Using a mandoline or V-slicer, cut the fennel into very thin slices. Place the fennel and lemon juice in a small bowl; toss to coat well.
6. Serve stew, discarding any mussels or clams that have not opened. Top with the fennel mixture and reserved fennel fronds.

TIPS

- Store mussels in the refrigerator and cook within 1–2 days. Keep them well drained. Discard any mussels that are open or smell bad, as well as any with cracked or broken shells.
- For wide orange strips, use a vegetable peeler to peel strips and avoid taking off too much of the white pith with the rind, as it's bitter.

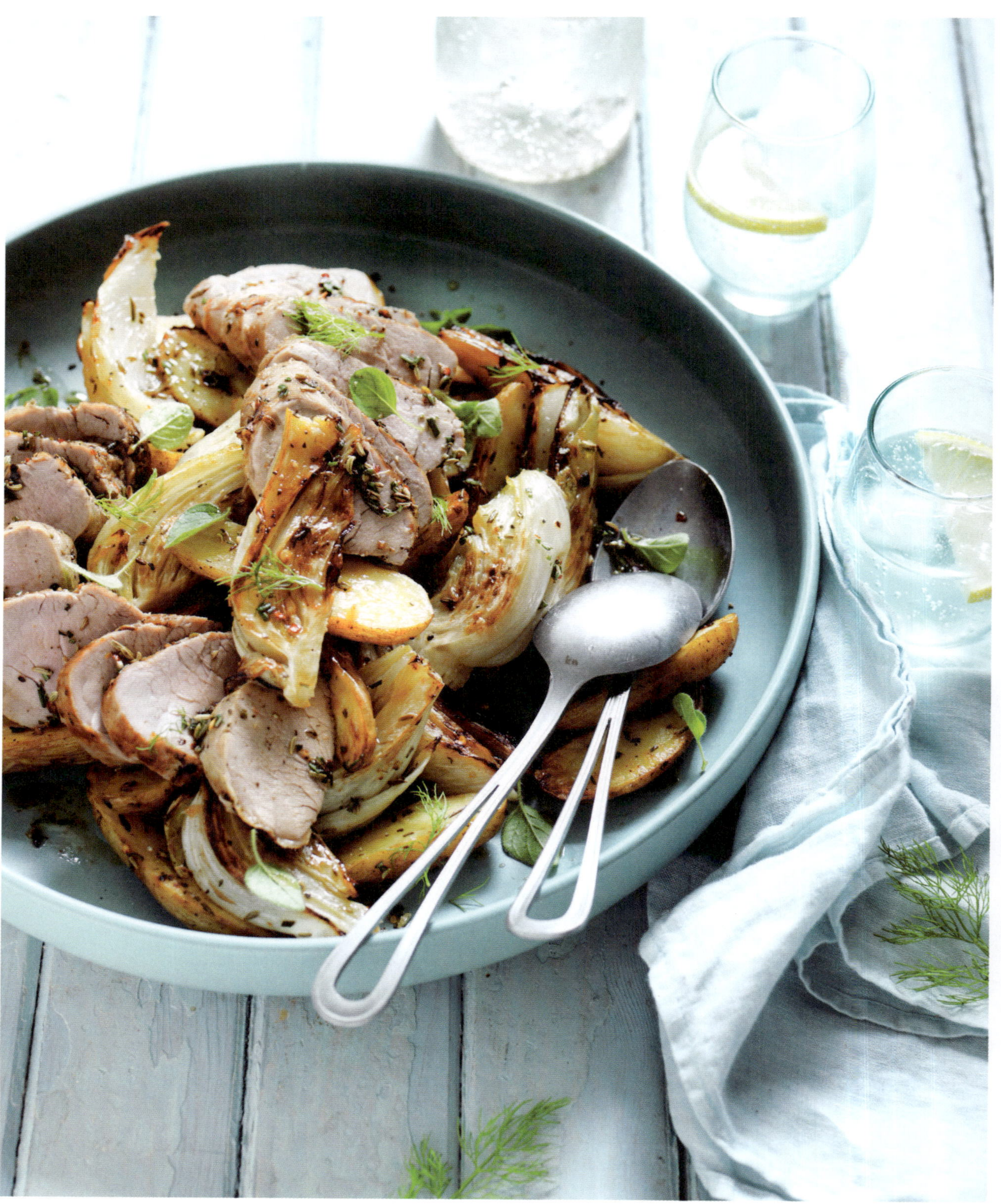

Roasted rosemary pork, fennel, and potatoes

PREP + COOK TIME **1 HOUR 15 MINUTES + STANDING** | SERVES **4**

Fennel can be roasted, sautéed, or eaten raw in salads. It can be fried as an accompaniment, or used as an ingredient in soups and sauces. It is also the name given to the dried seeds of the plant, which have a stronger licorice flavor. The Greek name for fennel is *marathon* and the place of the famous battle of Marathon literally means a plain with fennel.

1 tbsp finely chopped fresh rosemary leaves
2 tsp finely chopped fresh oregano leaves
2 tsp fennel seeds
1/2 tsp dried chile flakes
1/3 cup olive oil, divided
salt and freshly ground black pepper
3 medium fennel bulbs, trimmed and cut into wedges
2lb (900g) fingerling potatoes, halved lengthwise
1lb (500g) pork tenderloin
lemon wedges, for serving

1. Preheat oven to 425°F (220°C).
2. In a small bowl, combine the rosemary, oregano, fennel seeds, chile, and 1/4 cup of the olive oil; season with salt and pepper.
3. In a large roasting pan, place the fennel bulbs and potatoes. Drizzle with two-thirds of the rosemary mixture; toss to combine. Roast for 30 minutes.
4. Rub the pork with the remaining rosemary mixture. Heat the remaining olive oil in a large skillet over high heat. Add the pork; cook, turning, for 5 minutes or until browned all over.
5. Stir the potato and fennel bulbs in the roasting pan; place the pork on top of the vegetables. Roast for 20 minutes or until pork reaches an internal temperature of 145°F (63°C). Remove the pork from the roasting pan and let rest, covered loosely with foil, for 5 minutes.
6. Cut the pork into slices; serve with the potato, fennel, and lemon wedges.

TIPS

- You could replace the pork with chicken breasts, adjusting the cooking time accordingly.
- Sprinkle with fennel fronds and fresh oregano leaves before serving, if you like.

Mussels in chili broth with freekeh

PESCATARIAN | PREP + COOK TIME **1 HOUR 35 MINUTES** | SERVES **4**

Once you get the hang of working with mussels, you'll find they're easy to cook with and quite versatile. In this recipe, they soak in a rich chili broth, but mussels can be equally delicious in a simple white wine broth. They are also relatively low in calories and fat, all while being high in protein, vitamins, and minerals.

- 2lb (1kg) fresh mussels
- 1 cup dry white wine
- 1 tbsp olive oil
- 1 medium onion, finely chopped
- 2 stalks celery, trimmed, halved lengthwise, thinly sliced
- ½ lb (225g) carrots, peeled, trimmed, thinly sliced on the diagonal
- 2 tbsp tomato paste
- 1 cup cracked wheat freekeh (see tip)
- ½ tsp dried chile flakes
- 3 cups fish stock
- coarsely chopped fresh Italian parsley, to garnish
- lemon wedges, for serving

1. Scrub the mussels; remove beards. Discard any with broken or cracked shells, and any that are open and don't close when tapped.
2. Bring the wine to a boil in a large saucepan over medium-high heat. Add the mussels; cook, covered, for 8 minutes or until the mussels open. Drain the mussels in a colander over a large heat-resistant bowl; reserve the cooking liquid. Discard any that didn't open. Cover the mussels loosely with foil to keep them warm.
3. Heat the olive oil in the same pan over medium heat; cook the onion, celery, and carrot for 3 minutes or until the onion softens. Add the tomato paste, freekeh, and chile flakes; cook, stirring, for 1 minute or until fragrant. Add the stock and reserved cooking liquid; bring to a boil. Reduce heat to low; cook, partially covered, for 1 hour until the freekeh is tender.
4. Add the mussels to the pan; cook for 2 minutes or until heated through.
5. Top the mussel and freekeh mixture with parsley; serve with lemon wedges.

TIP

Freekeh is an ancient grain food made from roasted young green wheat; it is available at organic markets and some gourmet groceries.

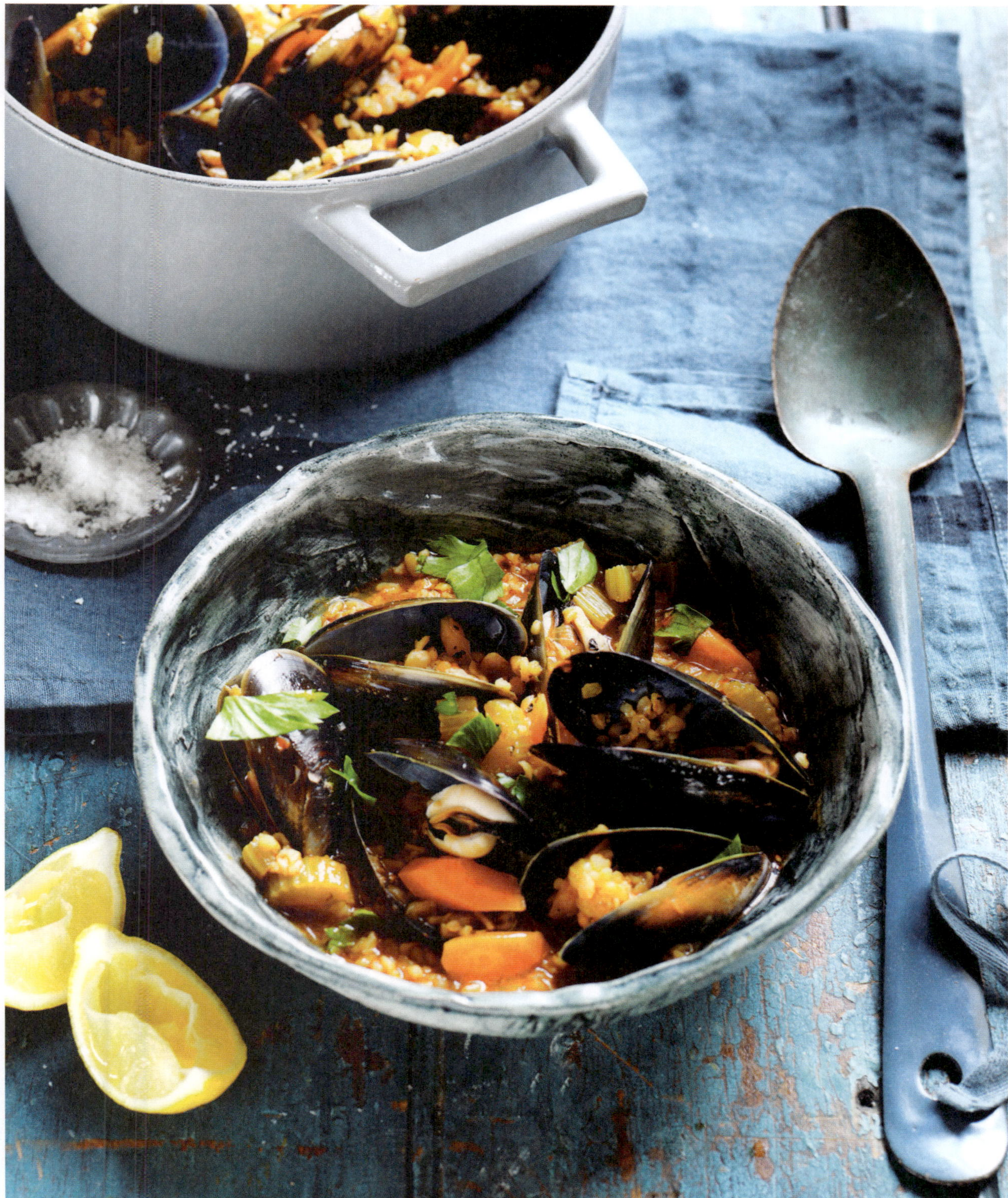

Baked salmon with tabouleh and tahini sauce

PESCATARIAN | PREP + COOK TIME **50 MINUTES** | SERVES **4**

Sumac adds a tart, lemony flavor to dishes, making it a perfect pairing with fish. The Romans used this ground spice as a sour element in cooking before lemons were introduced to their culinary world. It also goes well with chicken and meat, sprinkled on vegetables, or in a salad dressing—any foods you would ordinarily match with a fresh citrus flavor.

2lb (1kg) piece of skinless, boneless salmon fillet
1½ tsp sumac, divided
2 tbsp olive oil
salt and freshly ground black pepper
lemon wedges, to serve

tabouleh
1 cup small fresh Italian parsley leaves
¼ cup small fresh mint leaves
2 spring onions, thinly sliced
½ cup bulgur
10oz (283g) mixed cherry tomatoes
1 tbsp lemon juice

tahini sauce
½ cup Greek yogurt
1½ tbsp tahini
1 garlic clove, crushed
2 tsp lemon juice

1. To make the tabouleh, combine the herbs and spring onion in a large bowl; reserve half the mixture for serving. Bring the bulgur and 1½ cups of water to a boil in a small saucepan; reduce heat to low. Cook for 20 minutes or until tender; drain. Transfer the bulgur to a large bowl; add the tomato and lemon juice. Toss gently to combine; season with salt and pepper to taste.
2. To make the tahini sauce, whisk the ingredients in a small bowl until combined; season with salt and pepper to taste.
3. Preheat oven to 400°F (200°C).
4. Line a large baking sheet with parchment paper. Place the salmon on the baking sheet; sprinkle with 1 tsp of the sumac, then drizzle with the olive oil. Season with salt and pepper. Bake for 20 minutes or until the salmon is almost cooked through.
5. Top the baked salmon with the reserved herb mixture and remaining sumac; serve with the tabouleh, tahini sauce, and lemon wedges.

TIPS

- If fresh tomatoes from the garden are in season, use ½lb of small heirlooms, if preferred.
- You can make the tabouleh and tahini sauce several hours ahead; refrigerate, covered, until ready to use.

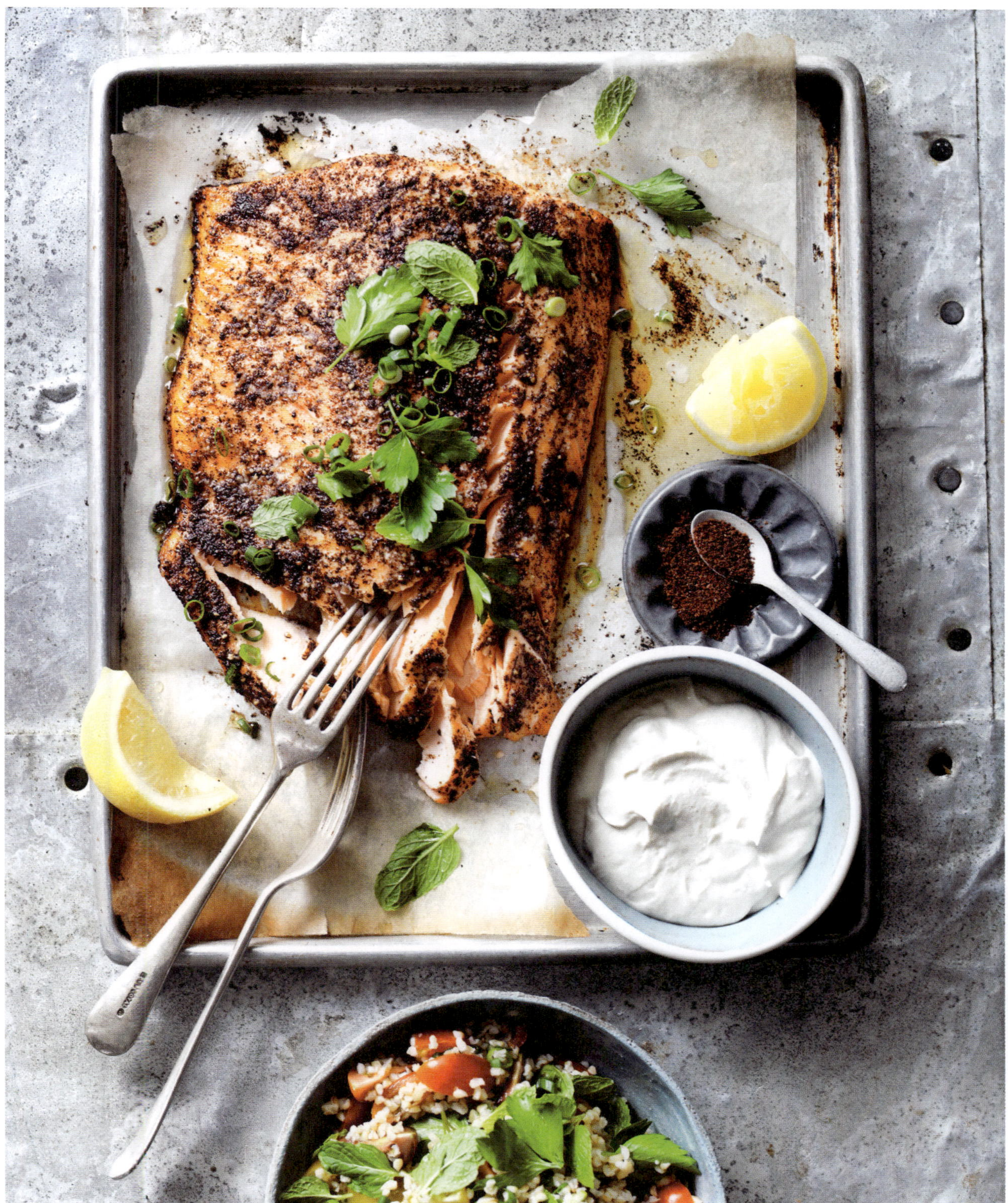

Almond gremolata roast chicken

PREP + COOK TIME **2 HOURS** | SERVES **4**

Gremolata is a versatile condiment and garnish sprinkled on a dish just before serving. Once it's warmed by the dish, the scent of the combined ingredients excites the palate. It's originally based on garlic, lemon rind, and parsley, but many variations exist using other ingredients. We've added roasted almonds for flavor and crunch.

$^1/_2$ cup roasted almonds, chopped
4 fresh sage leaves
1 tsp finely grated lemon zest (see tip)
2 garlic cloves, coarsely chopped
$^1/_3$ cup olive oil, divided
salt and freshly ground black pepper
4lb (1.8kg) whole chicken
4 stalks celery, plus pale inner leaves from the bunch
$^1/_4$ loaf sourdough bread, torn into 1$^1/_2$in (4cm) pieces
2 medium parsnips, peeled, trimmed, and cut into 1in (2.5cm) pieces
1lb (450g) rainbow baby carrots, trimmed, halved lengthwise
1 cup chicken stock

almond gremolata

$^1/_2$ cup finely chopped roasted almonds
1 small garlic clove, crushed
3 tsp finely grated lemon zest (see tip)
$^1/_3$ cup finely chopped fresh Italian parsley leaves

1. Preheat oven to 400°F (200°C). Oil two large roasting pans.
2. Blend or process the almonds, sage, lemon zest, garlic, and 1$^1/_2$ tbsp of olive oil until a rough paste forms; season with salt and pepper.
3. Pat the chicken dry with paper towel. Spread the almond mixture evenly between the chicken skin and breast and tops of the legs. Place the chicken in the oiled pan; season with salt and pepper.
4. Place the celery around the chicken; add the bread. Drizzle with another 1$^1/_2$ tbsp of the olive oil.
5. Place the parsnips, carrots, and stock in the other large roasting pan; drizzle with the remaining olive oil. Season with salt and pepper. Roast the chicken and vegetables for 1$^1/_4$ hours or until the chicken is cooked to an internal temperature of 165°F (75°C) at the thickest part of the thigh. Transfer the chicken, breast-side down, to a tray; cover loosely with foil. Let rest for 15 minutes.
6. Meanwhile, make the almond gremolata. Combine the ingredients in a small bowl; season with salt and pepper to taste.
7. Serve the chicken with the sourdough and vegetables, sprinkled with the almond gremolata.

TIP

Use orange zest instead of lemon zest in the chicken coating and gremolata, if you like.

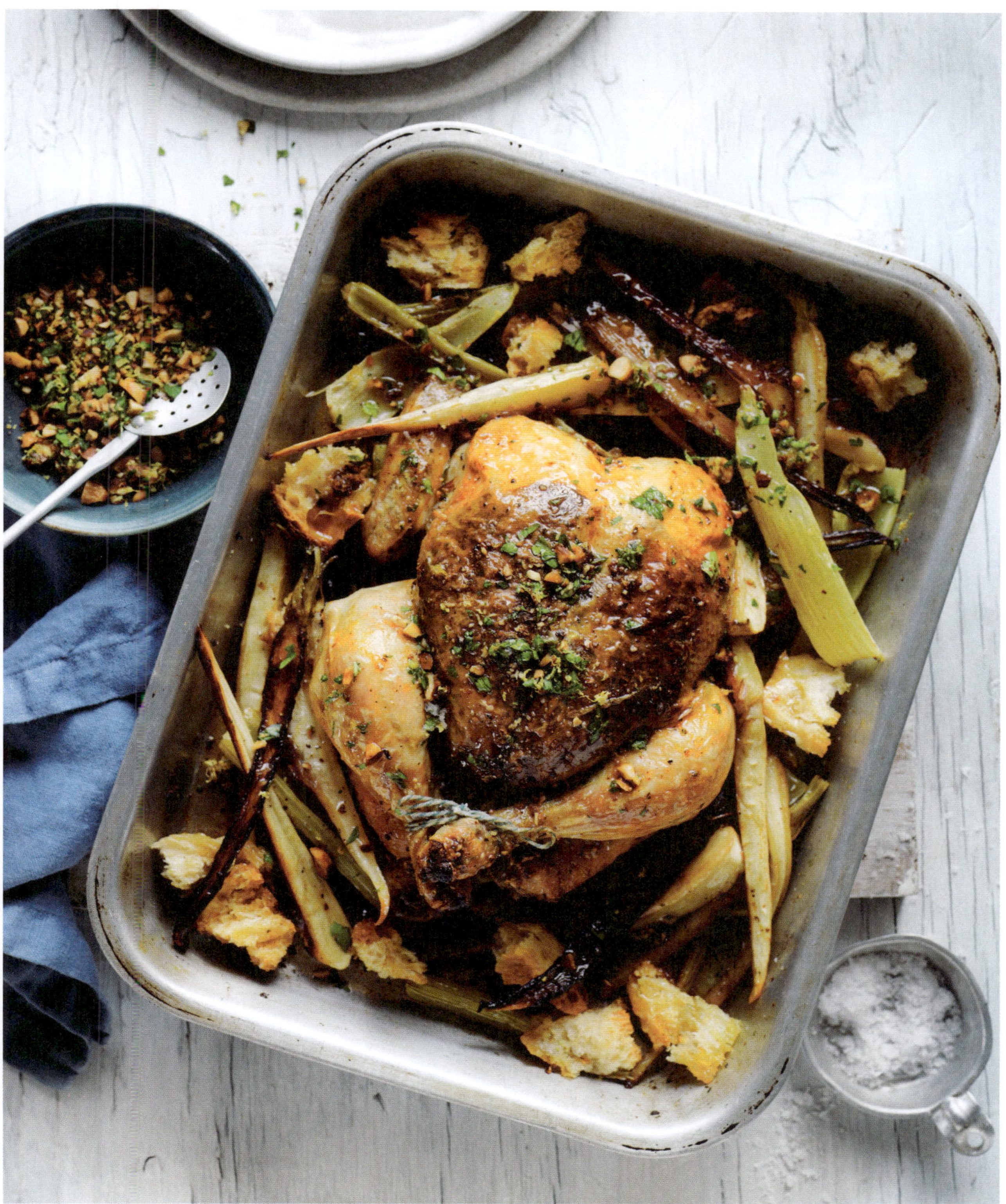

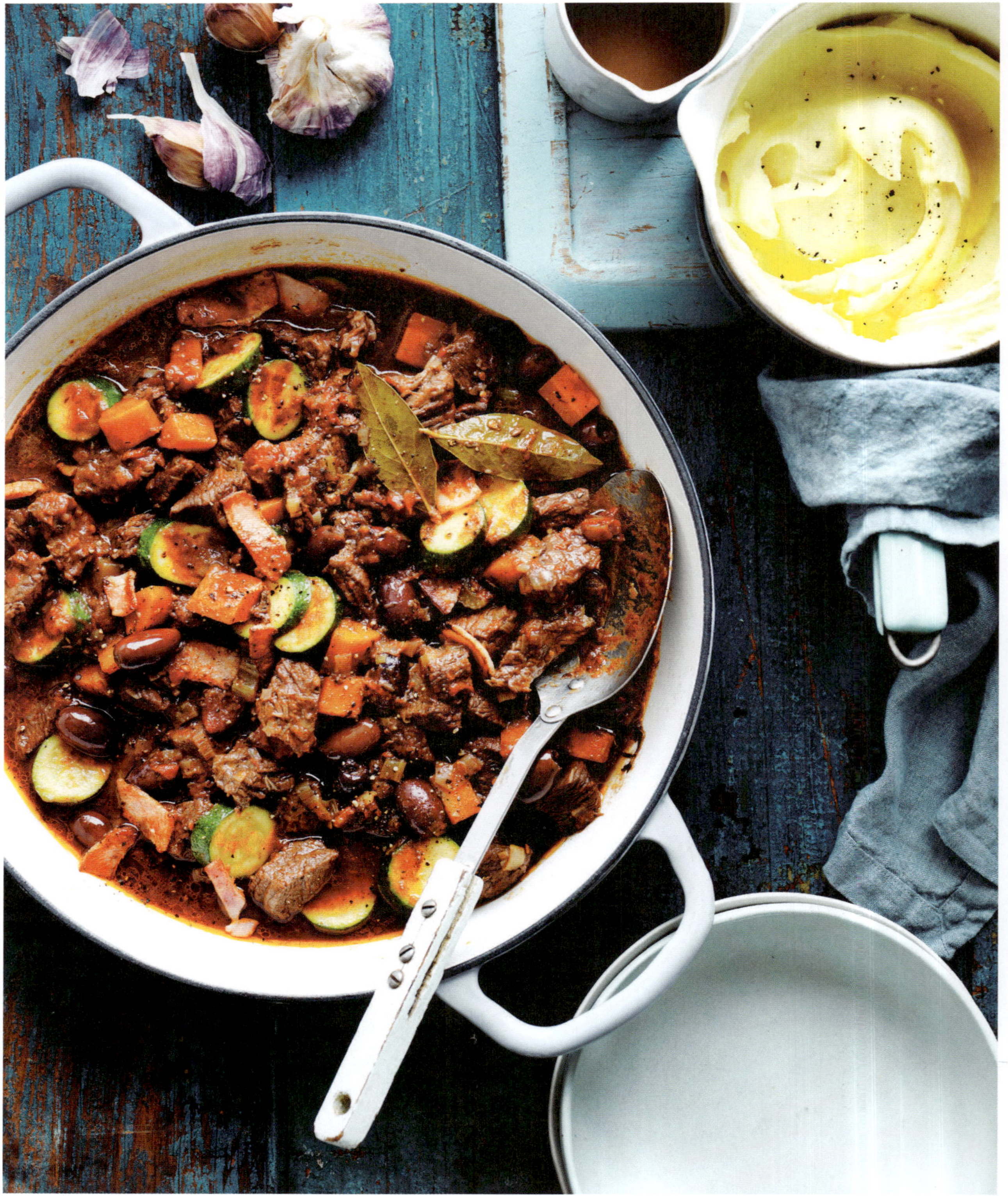

Provençale beef casserole

PREP + COOK TIME **1 HOURS 50 MINUTES** | SERVES **4**

If you wouldn't drink it, don't cook with it: that's the rule of thumb for choosing wine for cooking. A cheap wine of inferior quality will impart a less pleasant flavor than a great drinking wine. Serve a hearty casserole such as this one with mashed potatoes or crusty bread to mop up the sauce.

2 tbsp olive oil
2lbs (1kg) stewing beef, cut into ¾in (2cm) pieces (see tip)
4 slices bacon, roughly chopped
1 leek, thinly sliced
2 medium carrots, diced
2 celery stalks, trimmed, sliced thinly
2 garlic cloves, crushed
1 x 15oz (425g) can diced tomatoes
1½ cups beef stock
1 cup dry red wine
2 bay leaves
4 sprigs fresh thyme
6 sprigs fresh Italian parsley
2 zucchini, thickly sliced
½ cup pitted black olives

1 Heat the olive oil in a heavy-bottomed stockpot; sear the beef, in batches, until browned. Remove from the pan. Set aside.

2 In the same pan, cook the bacon. When cooked, remove to drain on a plate lined with a paper towel. Using the same pan with the bacon fat, cook the leek, carrots, celery, and garlic, stirring for 5 minutes or until the leek softens.

3 Return the beef to the pot, add the tomatoes, stock, wine, bay leaves, thyme, and parsley; bring to a boil. Reduce heat to low; cook, covered, for 1 hour, stirring occasionally.

4 Add the zucchini and olives; cook, covered, for 30 minutes or until the beef is tender. Remove and discard the thyme and parsley before serving.

TIP

Beef stew meat is usually chuck from the beef shoulder. You can also use beef short ribs or top and bottom round.

Seeded carrot and cabbage phyllo pie

VEGETARIAN | PREP + COOK TIME **1 HOUR + COOLING** | SERVES **6**

Seeds and nuts are little nutritional powerhouses. Walnuts in particular offer an array of antioxidant and anti-inflammatory nutrients, as well as valuable monosaturated and omega-3 fatty acids. Roasting seeds and nuts amplifies their flavor and, if they're a little on the stale side, it will freshen them up.

1/2 cup olive oil
2 leeks, white part only, thinly sliced
3 garlic cloves, crushed
2 tsp caraway seeds
3 medium carrots, coarsely grated
3/4 lb (375g) Napa cabbage, shredded
1/3 cup currants
1/3 cup finely chopped fresh mint
14 sheets phyllo pastry

seed topping

1/4 cup pumpkin seeds
1/4 cup slivered almonds
1/4 cup coarsely chopped walnuts
1 tbsp poppy seeds
1 tbsp sesame seeds

herb salad

1 medium cucumber
1/2 cup fresh Italian parsley leaves
1/2 cup fresh curly parsley leaves
1/4 cup fresh mint leaves
1/4 cup fresh dill
2 spring onions, thinly sliced
1 tbsp red wine vinegar
2 tbsp olive oil
salt and freshly ground black pepper

1 Heat 1/3 cup of the olive oil in a large frying pan over medium heat; cook the leek, garlic, and caraway seeds for 5 minutes. Add the carrot; cook for 3 minutes. Add the cabbage; cook for 5 more minutes or until the vegetables are soft. Stir in the currants and mint. Cool.

2 Make the seed topping. Combine the ingredients in a small bowl.

3 Preheat oven to 350°F (180°C). Cut a parchment paper circle to fit the bottom of a 10in (25.5cm) springform pan.

4 Divide the filling into seven portions. Brush one sheet of pastry with a little of the olive oil; top with a second sheet. Keep the remaining sheets covered with parchment paper topped with a clean, damp kitchen towel to prevent them from drying out. Place one portion of the filling lengthwise, in a thin line, along the pastry edge; roll the pastry over the filling. Starting at the center of the springform pan, carefully form the pastry roll, seam-side down, into a coil. As you did with the first, roll the remaining pastry sheets with olive oil and filling, but join each roll to the end of the previous one with a little olive oil and coil it around until the bottom of the pan is covered. Brush the top with olive oil.

5 Bake the phyllo pie for 20 minutes. Cover the pie evenly with the seed topping; bake for an additional 10 minutes or until golden

6 Meanwhile, make the herb salad. Using a vegetable peeler, peel the cucumber into ribbons. Place the cucumber in a medium bowl, add the remaining ingredients; toss gently to combine. Season with salt and pepper to taste.

7 Serve the phyllo pie with the herb salad.

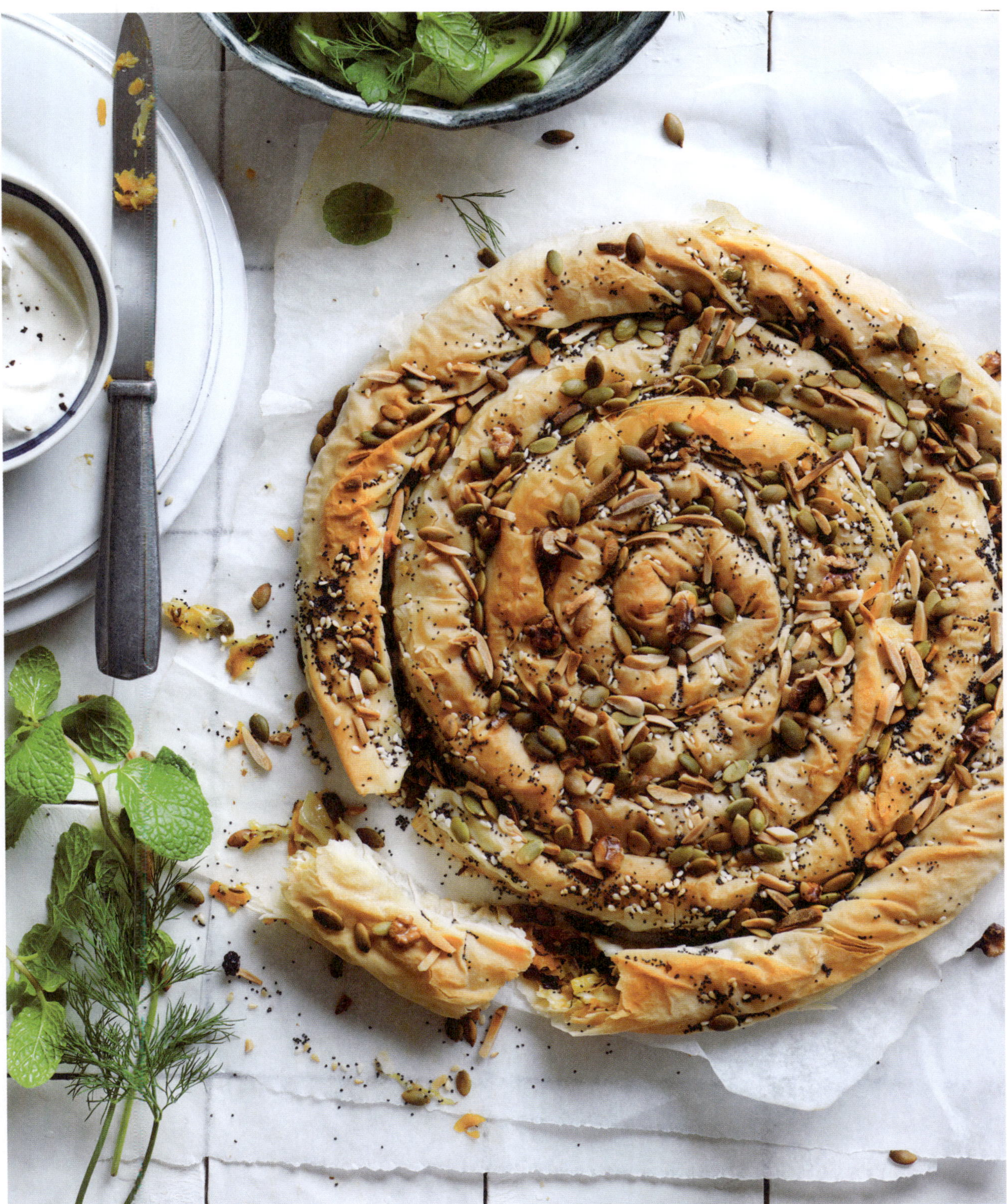

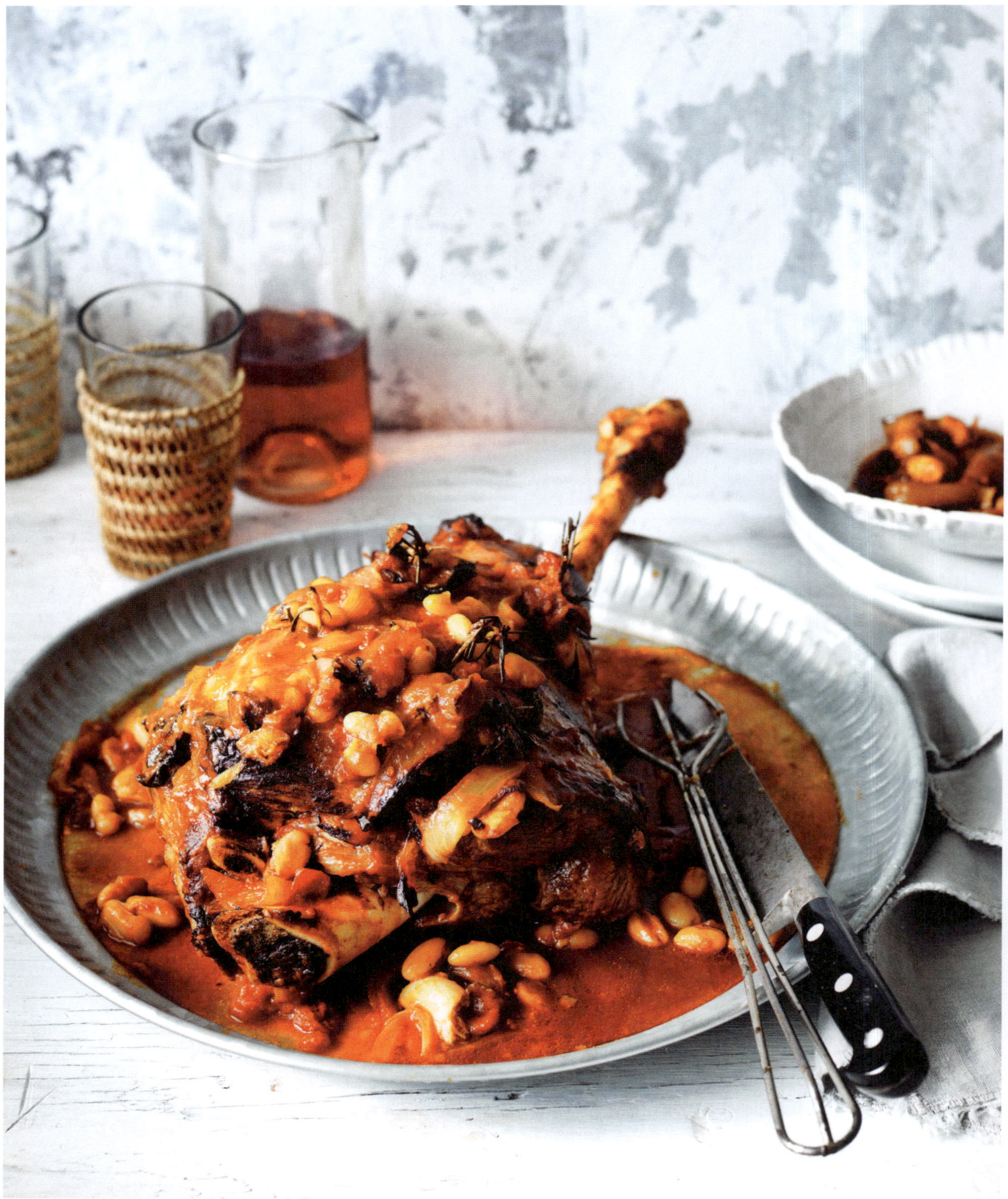

Roast lamb and beans

PREP + COOK TIME **2 HOURS 30 MINUTES** | SERVES **4**

Hearty and comforting, this French-style lamb roast will become a Sunday favorite. The leg of lamb is prepared in the classic way, pierced all over then studded with garlic and rosemary. Adding white beans, tomatoes, and stock gives it a twist from Brittany, a region in northwestern France. Serve with mashed potatoes and steamed green vegetables.

3½lb (1.5kg) leg of lamb, bone in (see tip)
1 garlic clove, thinly sliced
2 sprigs fresh rosemary
salt and freshly ground black pepper
1 tbsp olive oil
1 large onion, thinly sliced
3 garlic cloves, crushed
1 x 15oz (425g) can diced tomatoes
1 x 15oz (425g) can crushed tomatoes
2 cups beef stock
1 x 15oz (425g) can cannellini or Great Northern beans, drained, rinsed

1 Preheat oven to 350°F (180°C).

2 Trim the excess fat from the lamb. Pierce the lamb in several places with a sharp knife; press the sliced garlic and a little of the rosemary firmly into the cuts. Season the lamb with salt and pepper.

3 Heat the olive oil in an ovenproof casserole over medium heat; cook the onion and garlic, stirring, for 5 minutes or until the onion browns slightly. Stir in the diced tomatoes, crushed tomatoes, stock, beans, and remaining rosemary; bring to a boil.

4 Place the lamb, pierced-side down, on the bean mixture, cover; transfer to the oven. Cook for 1 hour. Uncover, turn the lamb carefully; cook, brushing occasionally with the tomato mixture, for 1 hour if you like it cooked medium, or until the lamb reaches an internal temperature of 145°F (63°C) for medium rare or 160°F (71°C) for medium.

TIP

You can instead use boneless leg of lamb or lamb shank, the meaty lower leg which is perfect for braising.

Black rice seafood paella

PESCATARIAN | PREP + COOK TIME **1 HOUR** | SERVES **6**

Short grain rice works best for paella. This version uses black "forbidden" rice, found at Asian markets and gourmet groceries, for its lovely nutty taste. If you don't have a paella pan or a heavy-bottomed frying pan large enough, use two smaller frying pans, as the mixture should only be about 1½in (4cm) deep.

1lb (450g) uncooked large shrimp
¼ cup olive oil
1 medium white onion, finely chopped
1½ tsp smoked paprika
1 red bell pepper, seeded, thickly sliced
2 garlic cloves, chopped
1 cup uncooked short grain black rice, rinsed
1 x 15oz (425g) can crushed tomatoes
2 cups vegetable stock
¾ lb (300g) skinless boneless firm white fish fillets, cut into 1½in (4cm) pieces
4 scallops on half shell (see tip)
¾ lb (320g) clams in the shell
salt and freshly ground black pepper
¼ cup fresh Italian parsley leaves
lemon wedges, to serve

1 Peel and devein the shrimp, leaving the tails intact.

2 Heat the olive oil in a large heavy-bottomed skillet or paella pan over medium heat; cook the onion, stirring, for 3 minutes or until softened. Add the paprika, red pepper, garlic, and rice; cook, stirring, for 2 minutes or until well combined. Add the tomatoes, stock, and 2 cups water; bring to a boil. Reduce heat to low; cook, stirring occasionally, for 40 minutes or until most of the liquid has been absorbed and the rice is tender.

3 Arrange the seafood on the rice mixture; season with salt and pepper. Cook over medium heat, covered, for 5 minutes or until the seafood is just cooked through. Don't worry if the rice seems dry and begins to form a crust on the pan. This crust is a mark of a good paella.

4 Serve the paella with parsley and lemon wedges.

TIP

Special order scallops on the half shell from your fishmonger. You may instead substitute ¼lb (100g) of bay scallops, if you like.

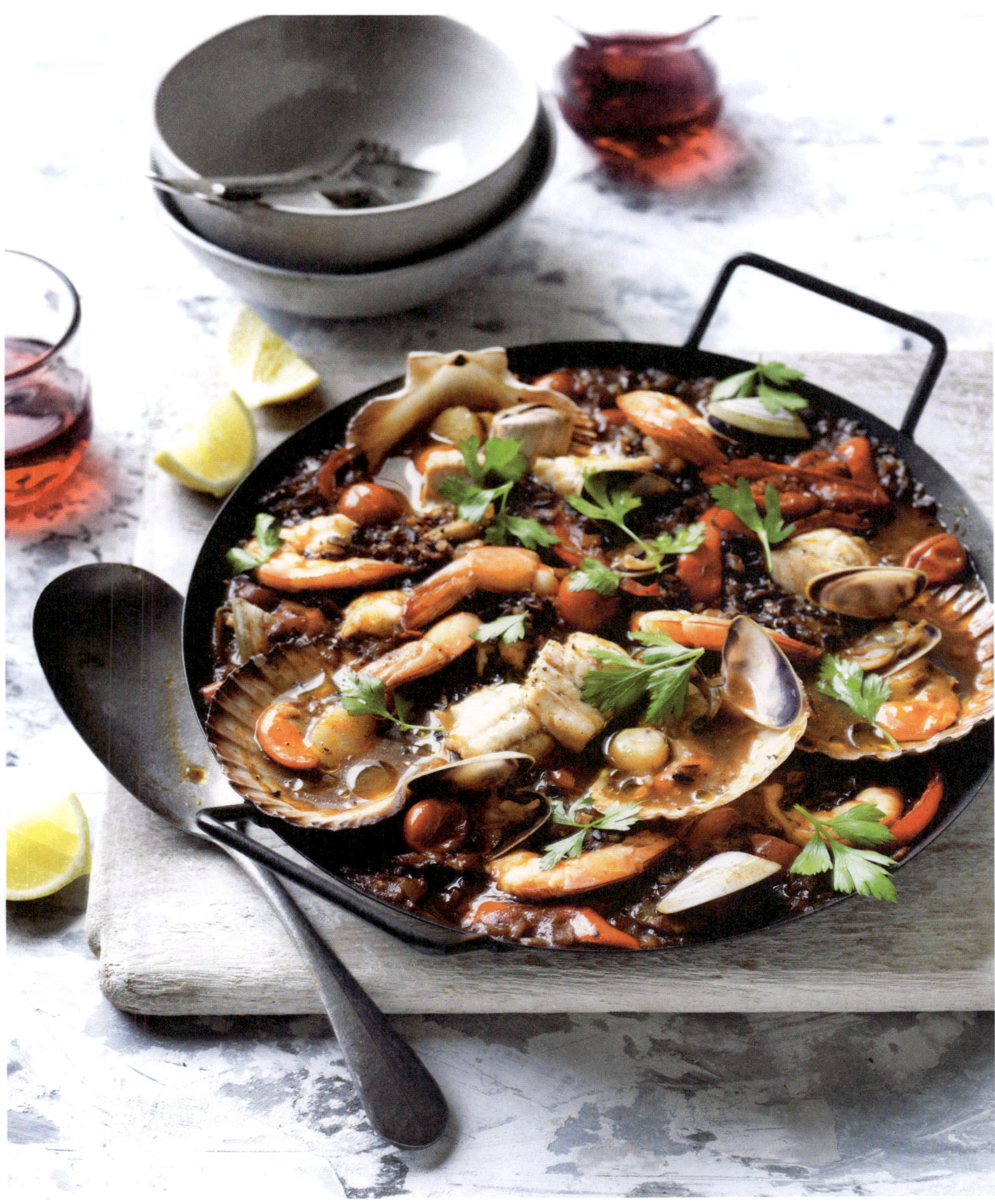

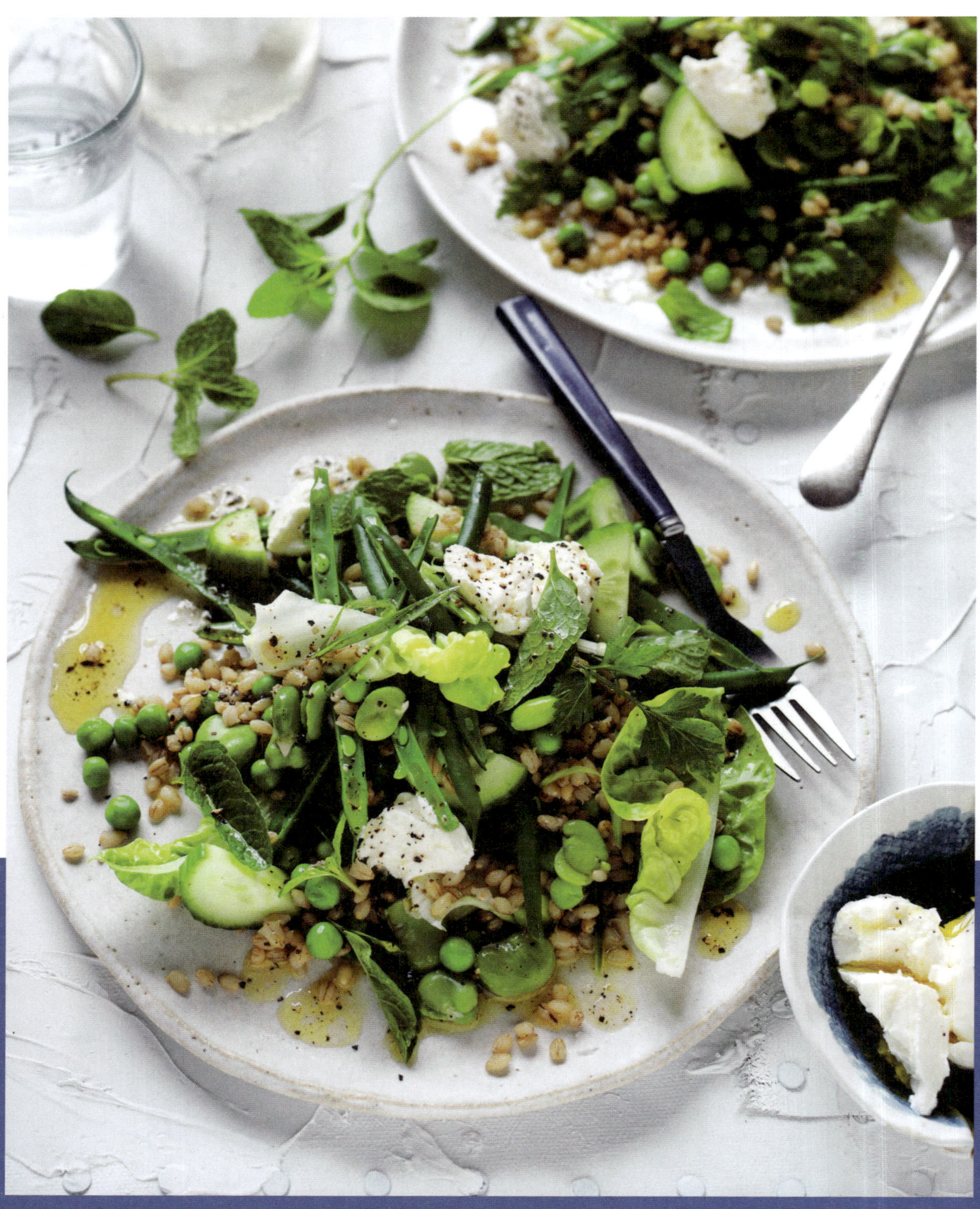

SALADS AND SIDES

From colorful salads packed with flavor and vibrancy to grains, fish, and delicious dips, these dishes are good enough to take center stage.

Squash fatteh with almond skordalia

VEGAN | PREP + COOK TIME **45 MINUTES** | SERVES **4**

Fatteh is an Arabic word meaning "crushed" or "crumbs." In a recipe it refers to fresh or toasted flatbread covered with other ingredients, such as the vegetables in this salad. You could make extra fatteh to use as an accompaniment for dip or salsa, serve as an appetizer for a shared meal, or nibble as a healthy snack.

2lb (900g) kabocha squash or butternut squash, peeled and seeds removed

1/4 cup olive oil, divided

1 1/2 tbsp za'atar, divided

salt and freshly ground black pepper

2 red bell peppers, seeded, thickly sliced

1 medium red onion, thickly sliced

1 large whole grain Lebanese bread round, split into two rounds (see tip)

1 1/4 cup canned chickpeas, drained, rinsed

2 tbsp pine nuts, toasted

1/3 cup fresh Italian parsley leaves

1/3 cup fresh mint leaves

lemon wedges, for serving

almond skordalia

1 cup blanched almonds

2 garlic cloves, crushed

1 cup coarsely chopped day-old bread

2 tbsp white wine vinegar

1/3 cup olive oil

1 Preheat oven 425°F (220°C). Line two large baking sheets with parchment paper.

2 Place the squash wedges on one baking sheet; drizzle with 1 tbsp of the olive oil and sprinkle with 1 tbsp of the za'atar; season with salt and pepper. Roast for 30 minutes or until just tender. Meanwhile, place the red pepper and onion on the second tray; drizzle with 1 tbsp of the olive oil. Season with salt and pepper; roast for 20 minutes or until tender.

3 Place the bread on a third, unlined, baking sheet, lightly brush with the remaining olive oil; season with salt and pepper. Toast the bread for 3 minutes or until crisp; cool. Break or tear into pieces.

4 Make the almond skordalia. Place the almonds in a heavy skillet; stir constantly over medium to high heat until they are browned evenly. Remove from the pan; cool. In the bowl of a food processor, combine the almonds, garlic, bread, and vinegar until wet breadcrumbs form. With the processor running, gradually add the olive oil in a thin, steady stream; add ½ cup water, pulse until the mixture is smooth. Season with salt and pepper to taste.

5 Place the vegetables, chickpeas, pine nuts, parsley, and mint on a platter; top with the remaining za'atar. Serve with the almond skordalia, toasted bread, and lemon wedges.

TIPS

- If you can't find Lebanese bread to purchase, use 4 pita bread rounds instead.
- You can assemble the salad ahead of time, omitting the bread. Serve bread on the salad, or on the side.

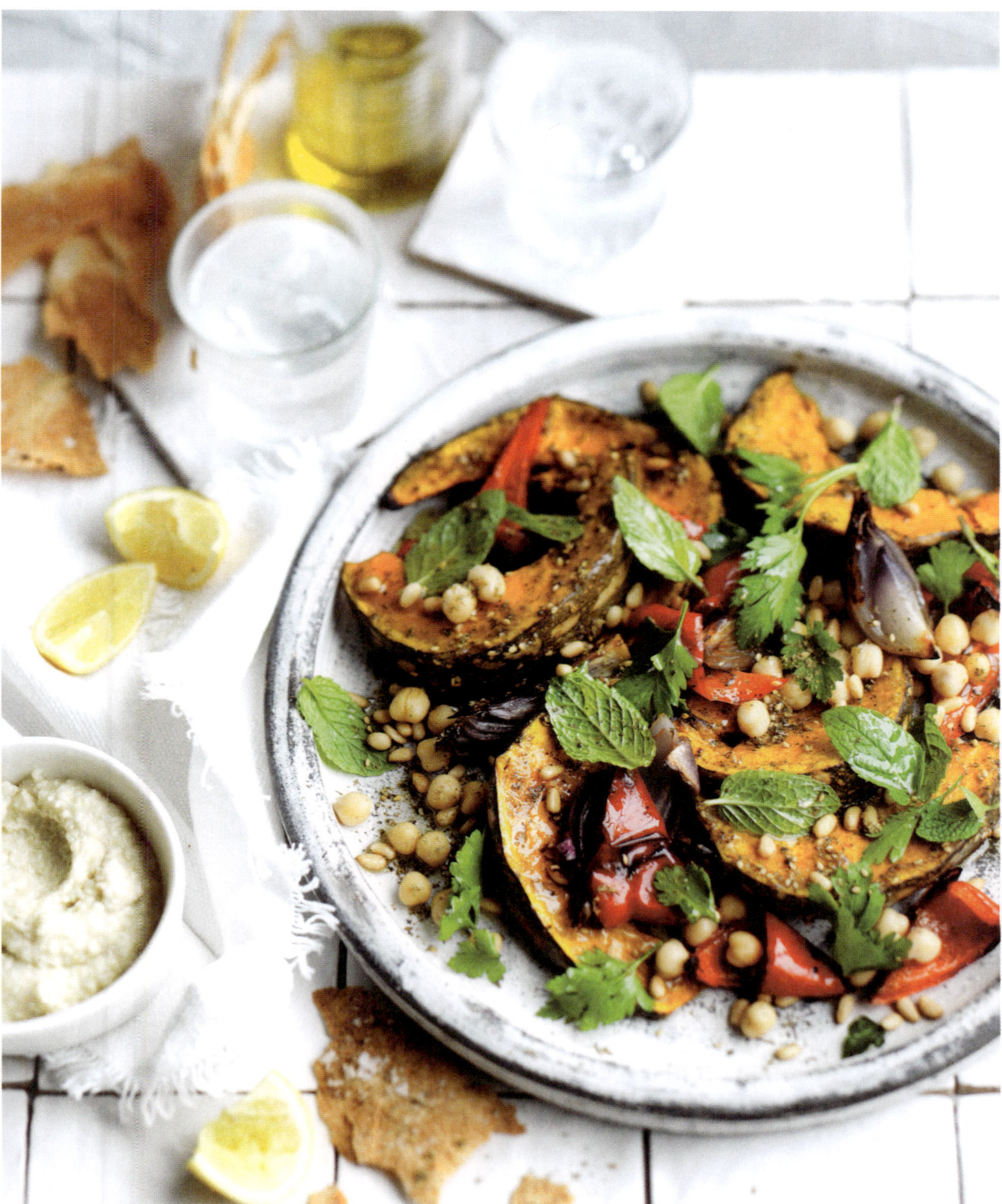

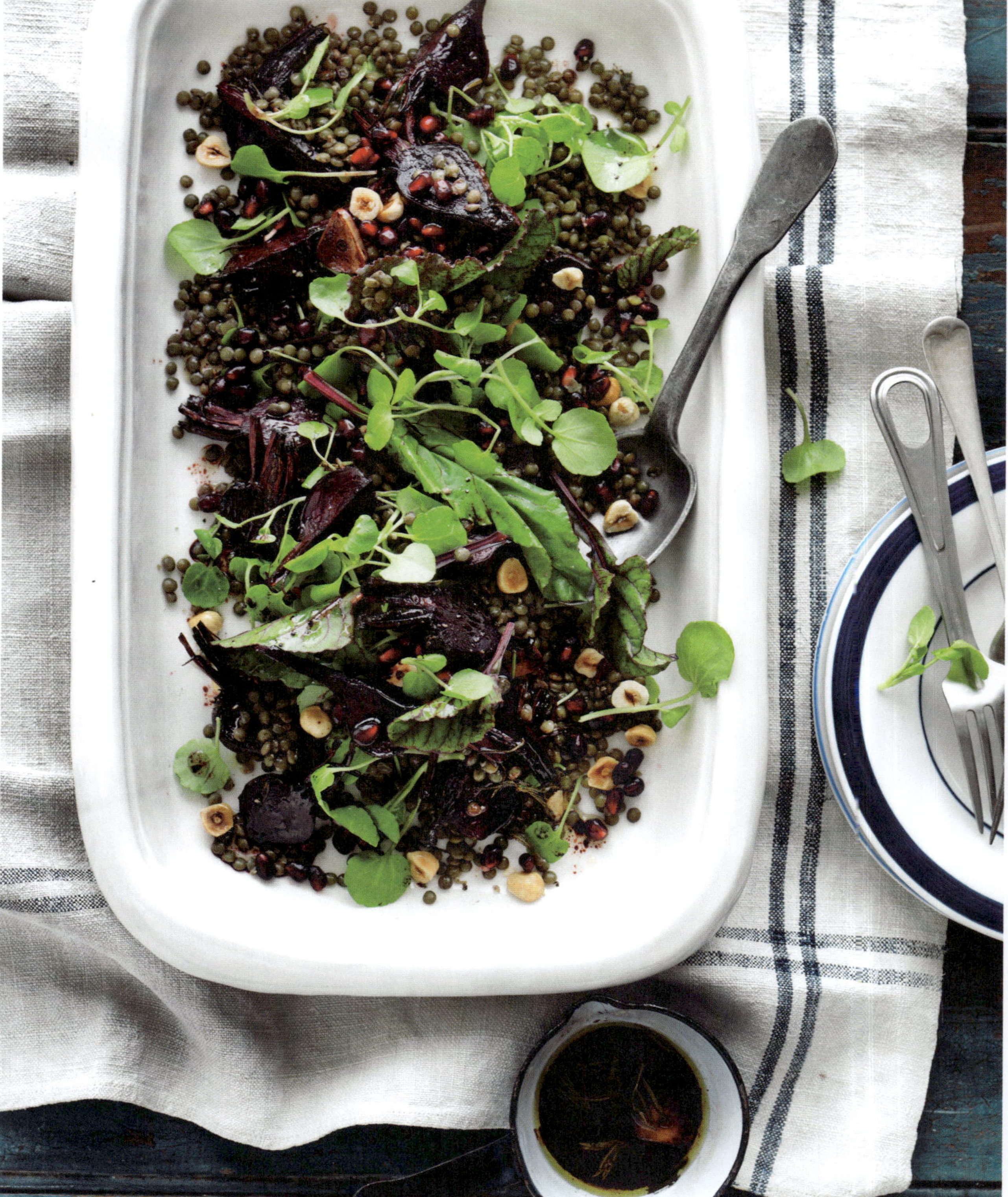

Beet, lentil, and arugula salad

VEGAN | PREP + COOK TIME **40 MINUTES** | SERVES **4**

French-style green lentils are closely related to the famous French lentils du Puy; these tiny green-blue lentils have a nutty, earthy flavor and a hardy nature that allows them to be rapidly cooked without disintegrating. If you can find fresh watercress, it's a delicious replacement for the arugula in this salad.

2lb (900g) small beets, stems and leaves attached
2 garlic cloves, sliced
1/4 cup fresh rosemary leaves
2 tbsp olive oil
1/4 cup balsamic vinegar
1/2 cup dried French-style green lentils, rinsed
3 cups arugula
1 cup of pomegranate seeds (see tip)
1/3 cup roasted hazelnuts, halved
salt and freshly ground black pepper

1. Preheat oven to 400°F (200°C).
2. Trim the beet tops to 1½in (4cm); reserve a few small leaves. Halve each beet (or quarter if large). Place the beets, garlic, and rosemary in a large heatproof casserole; drizzle with the olive oil and vinegar. Roast for 30 minutes or until tender.
3. Meanwhile, place the lentils in a medium saucepan; cover with water. Bring to a boil; cook the lentils for 25 minutes or until tender. Drain; rinse under cold water, drain.
4. Place the lentils, roasted beets and their cooking juices, arugula, half the pomegranate seeds, and half the hazelnuts in a large bowl; toss gently to combine. Season with salt and pepper to taste.
5. Transfer to a large bowl or platter; top with the remaining pomegranate seeds and hazelnuts, and the reserved beet leaves.

TIP

One pomegranate typically yields 1 cup seeds. To remove seeds from fruit, cut in half crosswise; hold a half, cut-side down, in palm, over a small bowl; hit the outside firmly with a wooden spoon. The seeds fall out easily; discard any white pith. Repeat with other half. (Or purchase already removed seeds.)

Roasted carrot, radish, and egg salad with romesco sauce

VEGETARIAN | PREP + COOK TIME **40 MINUTES** | SERVES **4**

Originating in the Catalonia area of Spain, romesco is a sauce consisting of blended almonds and red bell pepper. During the springtime, romesco is served as a dip for calçots, a spring onion native to Catalonia, which are roasted over an open fire until charred. Romesco is a great dairy-free alternative to creamy sauces and pesto.

2lb (900g) rainbow carrots, peeled, trimmed
1½ tbsp olive oil
salt and freshly ground black pepper
4 eggs
½lb (300g) small radishes, trimmed, halved
⅓ cup fresh Italian parsley leaves

romesco sauce
8oz (230g) jar roasted red peppers, drained
1 garlic clove, crushed
½ cup blanched almonds, roasted
2 tbsp sherry vinegar
1 tsp smoked paprika
2 tbsp chopped fresh Italian parsley leaves
⅓ cup olive oil

1. Preheat oven to 400°F (200°C). Line a large baking sheet with parchment paper.
2. Place carrots on the baking sheet, drizzle with olive oil; season with salt. Roast for 20 minutes or until tender and lightly browned.
3. Meanwhile, make the romesco sauce. In a food processor, combine the ingredients until smooth; season with salt and pepper to taste.
4. Place the eggs in a small saucepan, cover with cold water; bring to a boil. Cook for 2 minutes or until soft-boiled; drain. Rinse under cold water; drain. When cool enough to handle, peel the eggs; tear in half.
5. Place the carrots, radish, and eggs on a platter. Top with parsley; season with pepper. Serve with the romesco sauce.

TIP

Traditionally used to accompany fish, romesco sauce can also be paired with lamb or chicken, or served with crudités and crisp breads as a tasty dip.

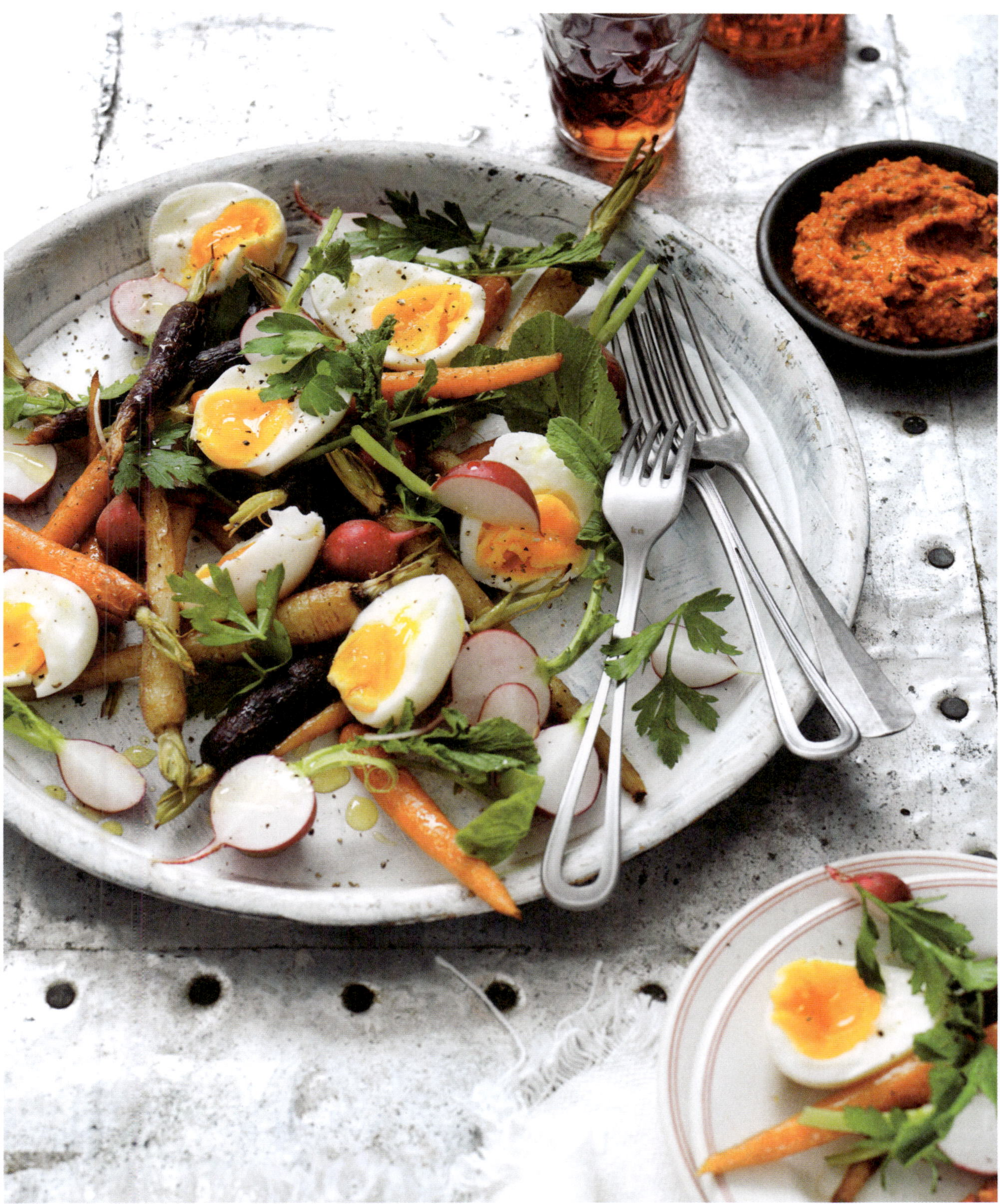

Roasted cauliflower, Tuscan kale, and spiced chickpeas

VEGAN | PREP + COOK TIME **40 MINUTES** | SERVES **4**

Chickpeas are an often overlooked legume full of protein, fiber, and folate. They are one of the oldest cultivated legumes in the world, with 7,500-year-old remains found in the Middle East. Chickpeas can be cooked and eaten cold in salads, ground into flour, fried as falafel, baked into a flatbread, used in stews, or blended to make hummus.

1 medium head of cauliflower, trimmed, cut into small florets

½ lb (220g) Brussels sprouts, trimmed, sliced

3 tbsp olive oil, divided

salt and freshly ground black pepper

1 x 15oz (400g) can chickpeas, drained, rinsed

1 tsp smoked paprika

1 tsp ground cumin

1 tsp ground coriander

1 bunch Tuscan kale (about 12 leaves), trimmed, torn

1 fresh long red chile, seeded, chopped finely

tahini dressing

1 tbsp tahini

1 tbsp pomegranate molasses (see tips)

1 small garlic clove, crushed

1. Preheat oven to 400°F (200°C). Line 2 baking sheets with parchment paper.
2. Place the cauliflower and Brussels sprouts on the baking sheet; drizzle with 1 tbsp of the olive oil. Season with salt and pepper; toss to coat in the oil. Place the chickpeas on another baking sheet; sprinkle with the paprika, cumin, and coriander. Season with salt and pepper; drizzle with another tbsp of the oil.
3. Roast the vegetables and chickpeas for 25 minutes. Massage the last tbsp of oil into the kale leaves until coated. Add the kale to the vegetables; roast for 5 more minutes or until the vegetables are tender and the chickpeas are crisp.
4. Meanwhile, make the tahini dressing. Combine the ingredients in a small bowl along with ¼ cup of water; season with salt and pepper to taste.
5. Drizzle the vegetables and chickpeas with the dressing and sprinkle with the chile; serve.

TIPS

- Pomegranate molasses is available from Middle Eastern food stores, major supermarkets, specialty food shops, and some delicatessens.
- This salad is best served either warm or room temperature.

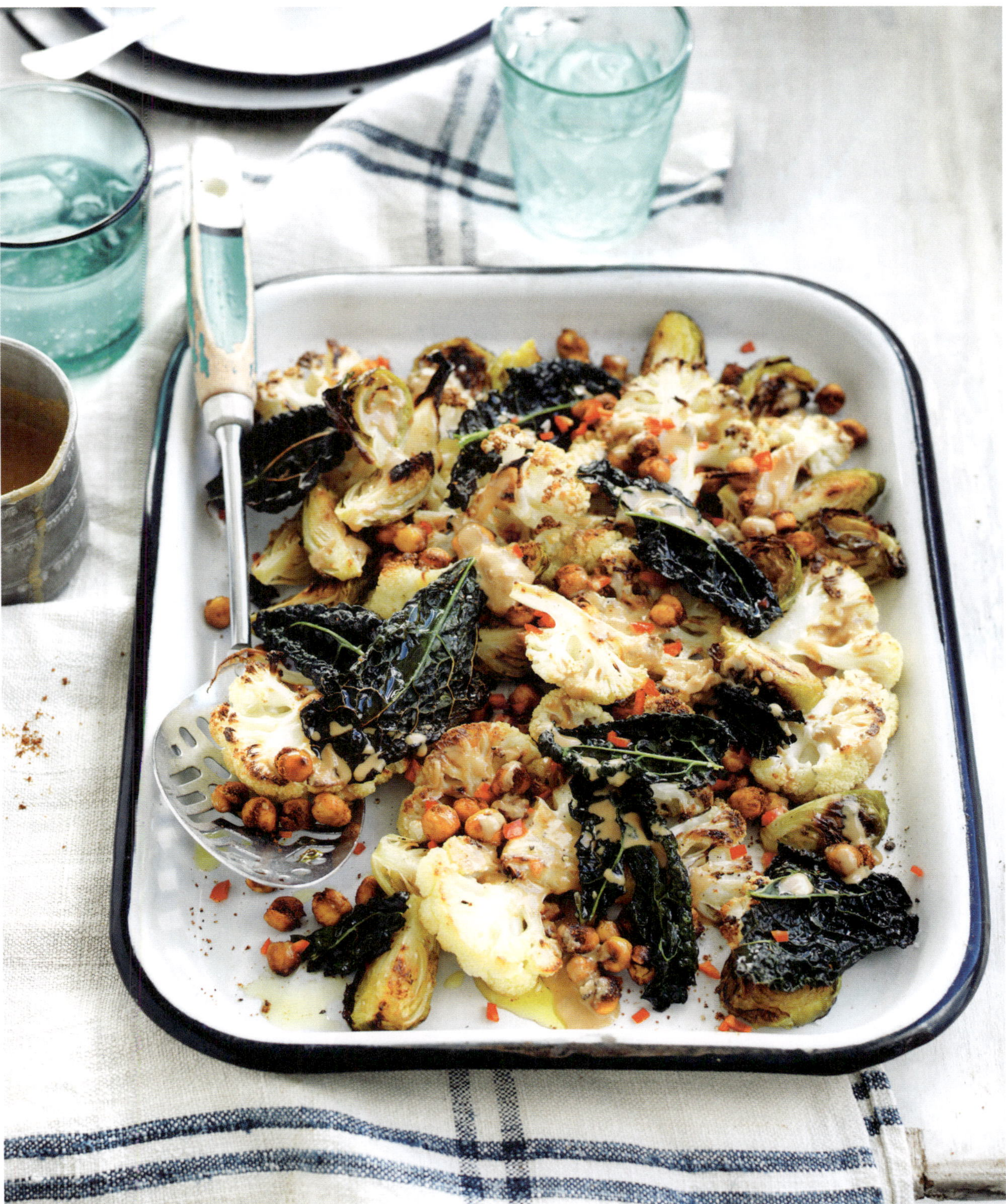

Chermoula tuna, chickpea, and fava bean salad

PESCATARIAN | PREP + COOK TIME **30 MINUTES + REFRIGERATION** | SERVES **2**

Traditionally used to flavor fish or seafood, chermoula is a spice marinade that contains as its core ingredients garlic, cumin, coriander, oil, and salt. You could make double the recipe and use it to dress other meats and vegetables, adding a fresh element to simple dishes. If the chermoula ingredients aren't blending well, add 1 tablespoon of water to the mixture.

$^{3}/_{4}$ lb (300g) piece tuna steak (see tips)
1 cup frozen fava beans
$^{1}/_{2}$ lb (225g) green beans, trimmed, halved lengthways
1 x 15oz (425g) can chickpeas, drained, rinsed
$^{1}/_{2}$ cup fresh Italian parsley leaves
1 medium lemon, segmented (see tips)
1 tbsp lemon juice
1 tbsp olive oil
lemon wedges, for serving

chermoula

$^{1}/_{2}$ small red onion, roughly chopped
1 garlic clove, peeled
1 cup fresh cilantro leaves, roughly chopped
1 cup fresh Italian parsley leaves, roughly chopped
1 tsp ground cumin
1 tsp smoked paprika
1 tbsp olive oil
salt and freshly ground black pepper

TIPS

- Purchase sashimi-grade tuna for this recipe. Alternatively, swap the tuna for salmon, if you like.
- To segment a lemon, use a small sharp knife to cut the top and bottom from the lemon. Cut off the rind with the white pith, following the curve of the fruit. Holding the lemon over a bowl, cut down both sides of the white membrane to release each segment.

1 Make the chermoula. In the bowl of a food processor, add all of the ingredients. Pulse until combined; season with salt and pepper to taste. Reserve three-quarters of the chermoula to serve.

2 Place the tuna in a shallow dish with the remaining chermoula; toss to coat. Cover; refrigerate for 30 minutes.

3 Meanwhile, cook the fava beans and green beans in a large saucepan of boiling water for 3 minutes or until just tender; drain. Place under cold running water to stop the cooking; drain well. Separate the fava beans; remove the gray skins from the fava beans.

4 Cook the tuna on a heated grill (barbecue) or ridged grill pan over medium heat for 2 minutes each side or until slightly charred on the outside but still rare in the center; remove the tuna to a plate, let stand for 5 minutes. Cut the tuna, across the grain, into slices.

5 Combine the fava beans, green beans, chickpeas, parsley and lemon segments in a medium bowl with the combined lemon juice and olive oil. Serve the tuna and salad topped with the reserved chermoula.

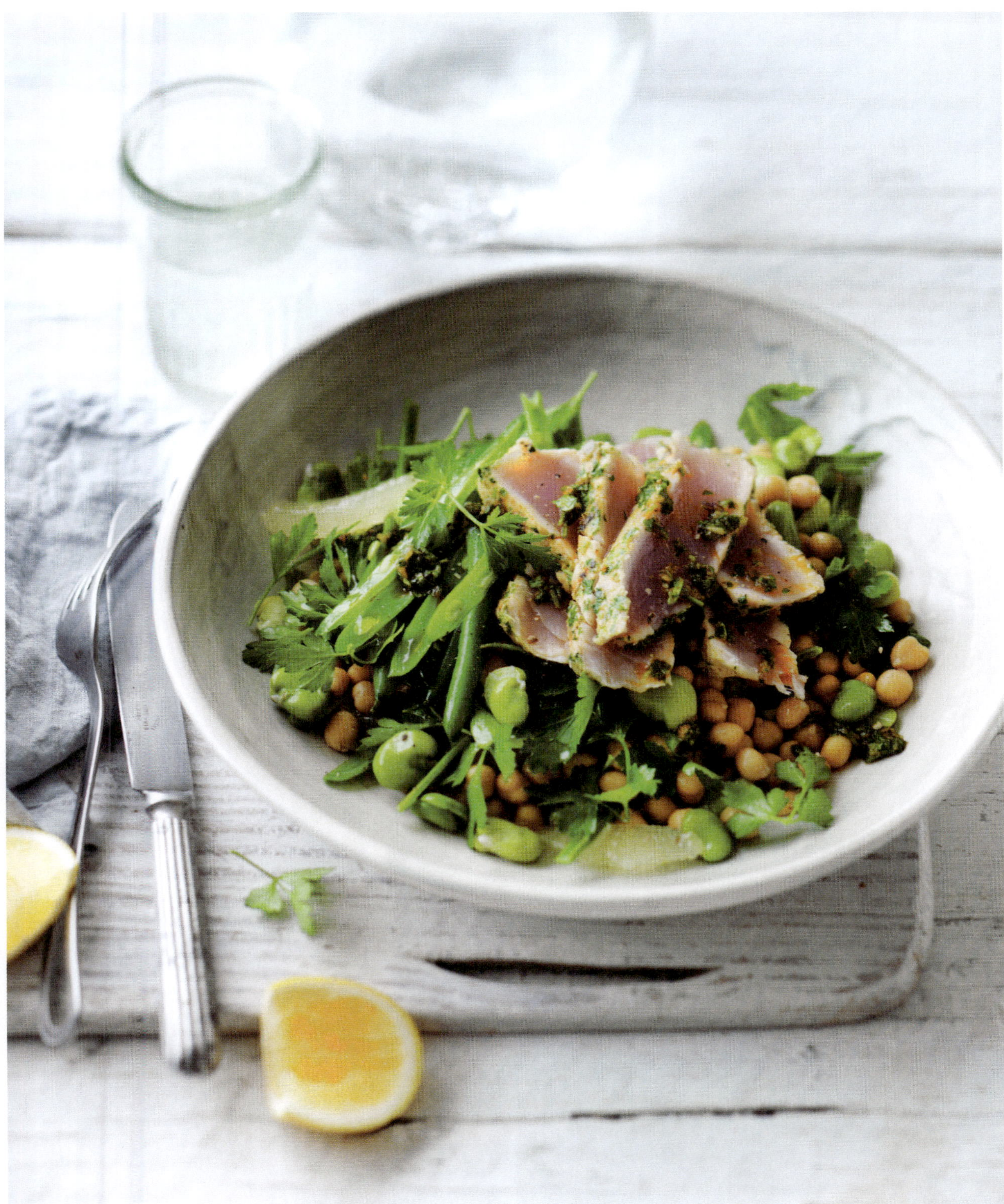

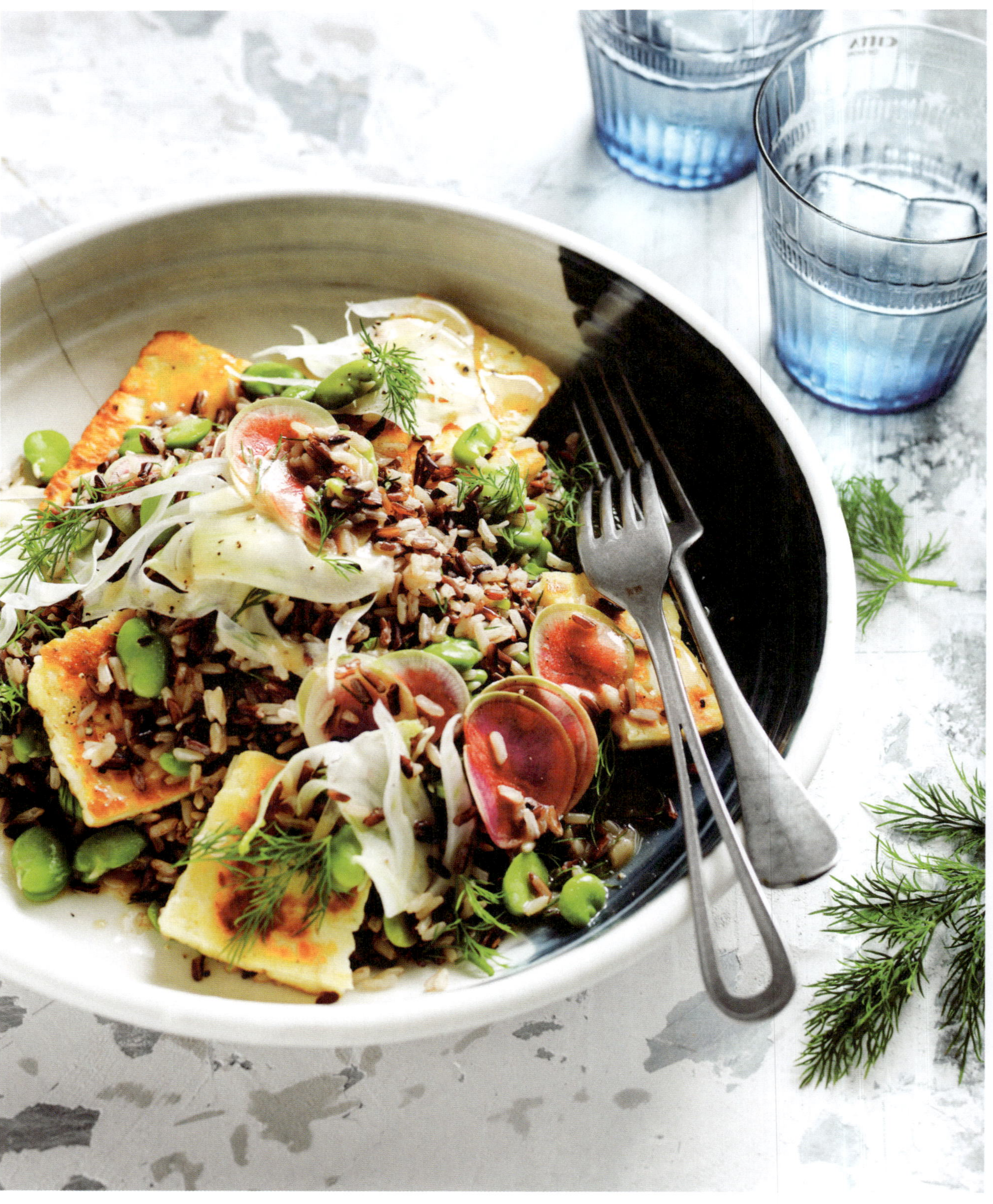

Mountain rice salad with halloumi cheese

VEGETARIAN | PREP + COOK TIME **50 MINUTES** | SERVES **4**

Halloumi is a Cypriot semi-hard, unripened brined cheese, often made from a mix of goat's and sheep's milk. Its high melting point allows it to hold its shape while being either fried or grilled. You shouldn't allow halloumi cheese to become cold after it's cooked—it becomes chewy and not nearly as delectable as when it's soft and golden, straight from the grill.

¼ cup red wine vinegar
1 tbsp Dijon mustard
¼ cup olive oil, divided
¼ cup honey
1 cup multicolor rice blend (see tips)
16oz (450g) frozen fava beans
1 baby fennel bulb, trimmed, thinly sliced
4oz (100g) radishes, thinly sliced
¼ cup fresh dill, roughly chopped
8oz (250g) halloumi cheese, cut into ½in (1cm) slices

1. Make the dressing. Place the red wine vinegar, mustard, 2 tbsp of olive oil, and 2 tbsp of honey in a screw-top jar; shake well. Season with salt and pepper to taste.
2. Cook the rice in a large saucepan of boiling water for 20 minutes or until tender; drain. Rinse under cold water; drain well.
3. Cook the fava beans in a large saucepan of boiling water for 3 minutes or until just tender; drain. Place under cold running water to stop the cooking, drain well; remove gray skins.
4. Place the rice in a large bowl with half the dressing; mix well. Add the fava beans, fennel, radishes, and dill; toss gently to combine.
5. Heat the remaining oil in a large nonstick frying pan over medium-high heat; cook the cheese for 1 minute on each side or until golden brown. Drizzle with the remaining honey.
6. Place the rice salad on a large platter; top with the halloumi and pan juices. Just before serving, drizzle with the remaining dressing.

TIPS

- You can find multicolor blends of white, brown, black, and red rice at most local gourmet groceries or organic supermarkets. They're sometimes called "royal rice" blends or "mountain rice" blends.
- You can use frozen peas instead of fava beans.
- Sprinkle with dill sprigs before serving, if you like.

Salade niçoise

PESCATARIAN | PREP + COOK TIME **45 MINUTES** | SERVES **4**

If you can't actually be living in the city of Nice, on the French Riviera, the very least you can do is enjoy some of the salad that originated there. Popularized by celebrity chefs, salade niçoise is now found all over the world. Like with all great dishes, there's much debate as to what ingredients should or should not go into it.

1½lb (600g) baby potatoes, halved
½lb (200g) green beans, trimmed, halved
3 eggs
2 x 6oz (200g) tuna steaks (see tips)
1 tbsp olive oil
salt and freshly ground black pepper
½ small red onion, thinly sliced
10oz (250g) cherry tomatoes, halved
⅓ cup pitted small black olives
⅓ cup caperberries, rinsed (see tips)
¼ cup small fresh basil leaves
2 tbsp fresh Italian parsley leaves, roughly chopped

dressing

2 tbsp olive oil
2 tbsp white wine vinegar
2 tsp lemon juice

1. Place the potatoes in a small saucepan, cover with cold water; bring to a boil. Cook for 15 minutes or until tender; drain.
2. Meanwhile, boil, steam, or microwave the beans until tender; drain. Place under cold running water to stop cooking; drain well.
3. To make the dressing, place the ingredients in a small screw-top jar; shake well. Season with salt and pepper to taste.
4. Place the hot potatoes in a large bowl with one-third of the dressing; toss gently to combine.
5. Place the eggs in a small saucepan, cover with cold water; bring to a boil. Cook for 2 minutes or until soft-boiled; drain. Rinse under cold water; drain. When the eggs are cool enough to handle, peel; tear in half.
6. Brush the tuna with olive oil; season with salt and pepper. Heat a large heavy-bottomed pan over high heat; cook the tuna for 1 minute on each side for medium-rare or until cooked as desired. Cut into thin slices.
7. Add the beans, onion, tomatoes, eggs, olives, caperberries, herbs, and the remaining dressing to the bowl; toss gently to combine. Serve topped with the tuna.

TIPS

- Instead of fresh tuna, use an equivalent amount of canned tuna in oil, if you like.
- Substitute regular capers for the caperberries, if you prefer.

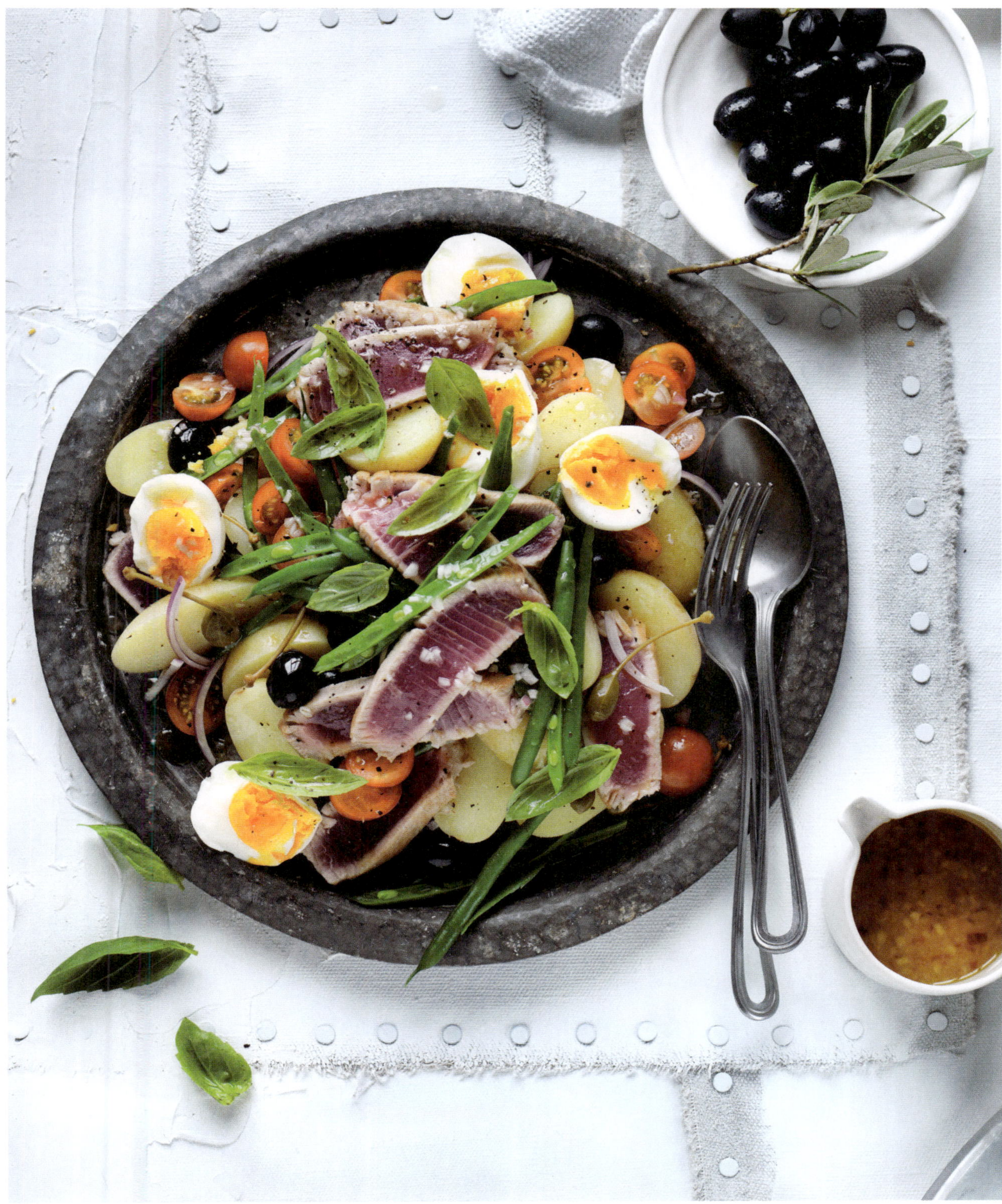

Grilled octopus

PESCATARIAN | PREP + COOK TIME **30 MINUTES + REFRIGERATION** | SERVES **4**

Like squid, octopus requires either long slow cooking (usually for larger mollusks) or quick cooking over high heat (usually for small mollusks)—anything in between will make it tough and rubbery. When grilling, make sure the grill is very hot before adding the baby octopus. You can sprinkle nasturtium leaves over the salad if you like.

3 medium lemons, divided
1/3 cup olive oil
1/2 tsp dried oregano leaves
2 garlic cloves, crushed
salt and freshly ground black pepper
2lb (1kg) fresh octopus, cleaned, cut into large pieces (see tips)
4 fresh long red chiles
1/2 cup arugula, to garnish
fresh Italian parsley leaves, to garnish

1. Make the dressing. Finely grate the zest from 1 lemon; squeeze out the juice. Place the zest, juice, olive oil, oregano, and garlic in a screw-top jar; shake well. Season with salt and pepper to taste.
2. Place the octopus pieces and half the dressing in a large bowl; toss to coat in the mixture. Cover; refrigerate for 30 minutes.
3. Preheat the grill (barbecue) or ridged grill pan on high. Cook the octopus over high heat for 6 minutes or until browned and tender. Remove from heat and cover loosely with foil.
4. Cut the remaining lemons in half crosswise; cook, cut-side down, on the heated grill (barbecue) or ridged grill pan for 2 minutes or until browned. Transfer to a plate. Cook the whole chiles for 4 minutes or until slightly blackened; slice thickly.
5. Combine the octopus with the remaining dressing and chile; top with arugula and parsley. Serve with the chargrilled lemons.

TIP

You may occasionally find octopus at the fish counter. Otherwise, special order it from your fishmonger. (Ask the staff to clean it.) If you use prepacked or frozen octopus, make sure it's uncooked.

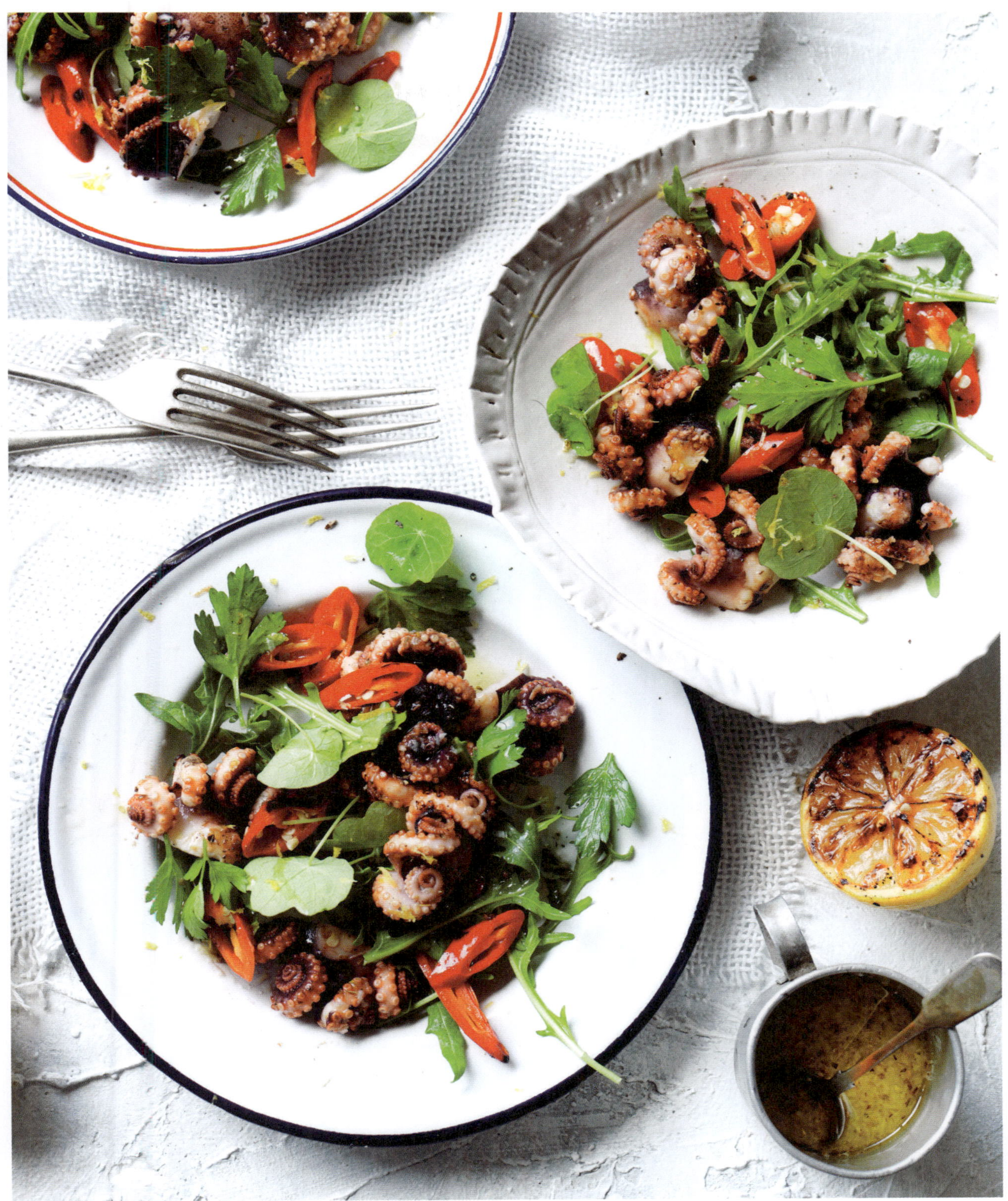

Delicious dips

Dips are great to serve at a party or as part of a mezze banquet. They're a communal affair as guests gather around and share in the delicious offerings. These Mediterranean dips work well with raw vegetables, pita bread, or served as accompaniments to a main meal.

Tzatziki

VEGETARIAN | PREP + COOK TIME **15 MINUTES + REFRIGERATION**
MAKES **$1^3/_4$ CUPS**

Place a cheesecloth-lined strainer over a bowl; spoon in 2 cups Greek yogurt and $^1/_2$ teaspoon of salt. Cover, refrigerate for 2 hours or until thickened; discard liquid. Meanwhile, combine 1 roughly grated medium cucumber and $^1/_2$ tsp of salt in a small bowl; let stand for 20 minutes. Squeeze out excess liquid from the cucumber. Combine the yogurt, cucumber, 1 crushed garlic clove, and 2 tbsp of chopped fresh mint leaves; season with salt and pepper to taste.

Lima bean hummus

VEGETARIAN | PREP + COOK TIME **10 MINUTES** | MAKES **3 CUPS**

Drain and rinse 2 x 15oz (425g) cans lima beans. Blend or process the beans with $^1/_2$ cup warm water, $^1/_4$ cup Greek yogurt, 2 tbsp of lemon juice, 3 tsp of ground cumin, 2 crushed garlic cloves, and $^1/_4$ cup tahini until smooth; season with salt and pepper to taste. Sprinkle with ground cumin to serve.

Taramasalata

PESCATARIAN | PREP TIME **25 MINUTES + REFRIGERATION**
MAKES **$1^2/_3$ CUPS**

Boil, steam, or microwave 1 roughly chopped large potato until tender. Refrigerate until cold. Mash the potato in a small bowl with 3oz (90g) salted fish roe (red or white), half of a finely grated small white onion, $^3/_4$ cup olive oil, $^1/_4$ cup white wine vinegar, and 1 tbsp of lemon juice until smooth. Season with pepper; serve drizzled with extra olive oil.

CLOCKWISE from top

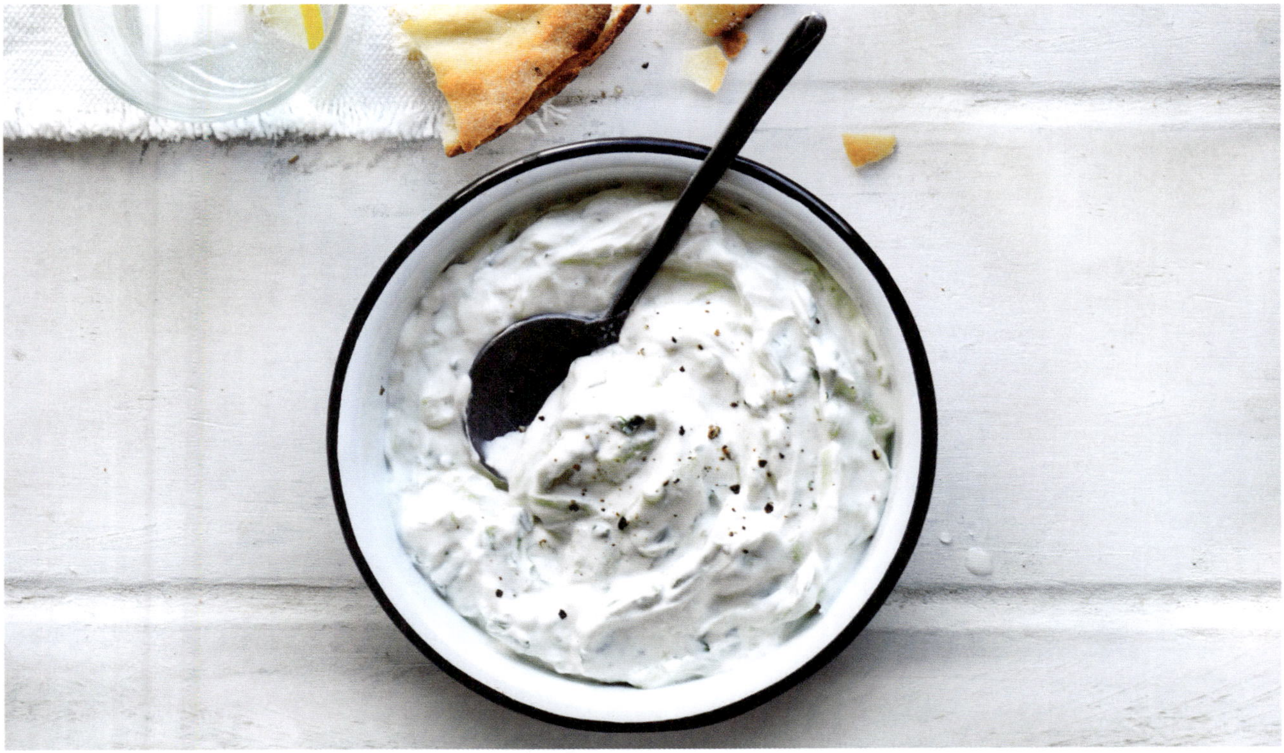

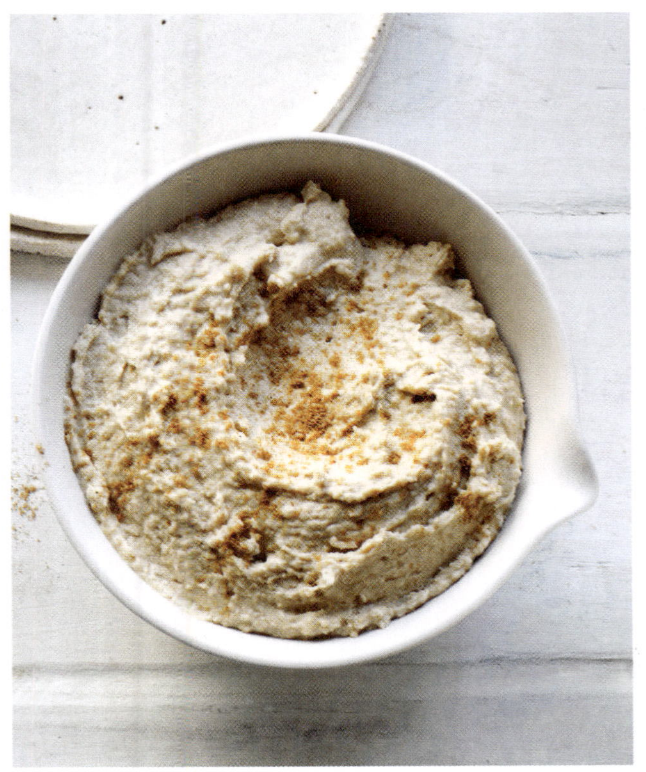

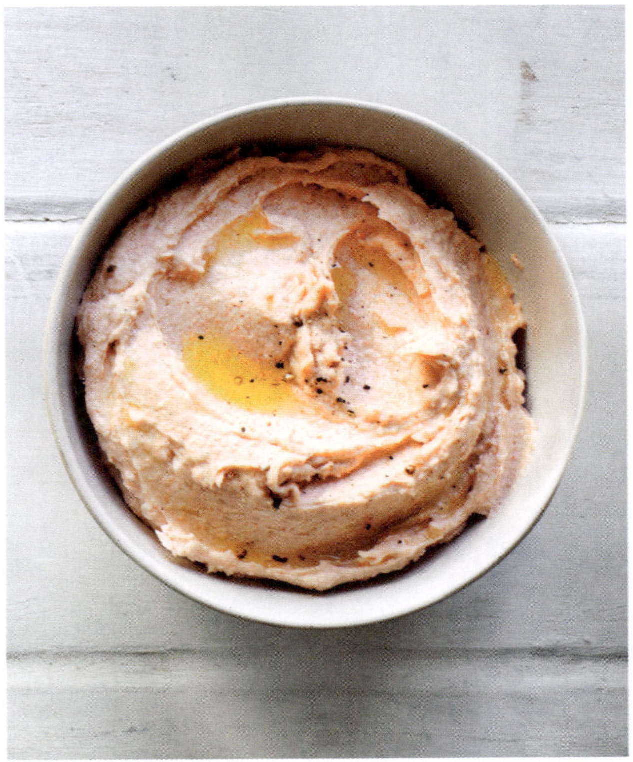

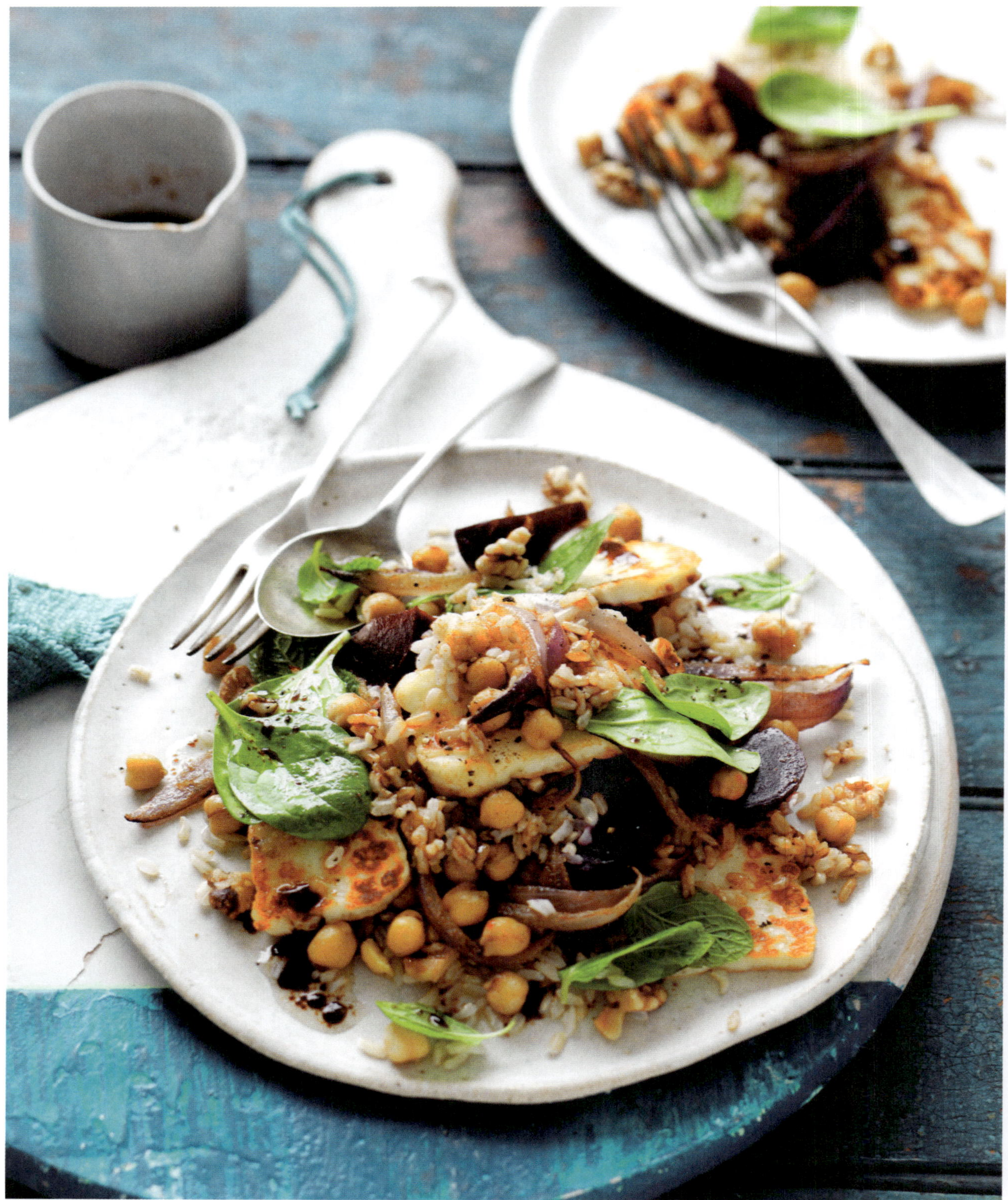

Beet, halloumi cheese, chickpea, and rice salad

VEGETARIAN | PREP + COOK TIME **30 MINUTES** | SERVES **4**

Canned chickpeas must be drained of their liquid before using. Empty the contents of the can into a strainer, allowing the liquid to drain away. Hold the strainer under cold running water and rinse the chickpeas. The chickpea liquid, called aquafaba, can be reserved and whipped into peaks like you would egg white, for a vegan-friendly meringue, pavlova, or mousse.

1 cup brown rice
1/3 cup olive oil, divided
1 small red onion, cut into wedges
1 tsp ground cumin
1 tsp ground coriander
15oz (425g) can chickpeas, drained, rinsed
1lb (500g) beets, cooked, quartered
3 cups spinach leaves
1 cup fresh mint leaves
1/2 cup walnuts, roasted, roughly chopped
2 tbsp balsamic vinegar, divided
salt and freshly ground black pepper
7oz (200g) halloumi cheese,
sliced into 1/4 in (0.5cm) slices (see tip)

1. Cook the rice in a large saucepan of boiling water for 25 minutes or until just tender; drain.
2. Meanwhile, heat 1 tbsp of olive oil in a large skillet over medium heat. Add the onion; cook, stirring, for 5 minutes or until tender. Add the cumin and coriander; cook, stirring, for 30 seconds or until fragrant. Add the chickpeas and beet; stir until heated through.
3. Combine 1 tbsp of balsamic vinegar and 2 tbsp of olive oil in a small jar with a screw top. Shake to combine. In a large bowl, combine the rice, spinach, mint, and walnuts. Add the beet-chickpea mixture and the balsamic dressing; toss gently. Season with salt and pepper.
4. Heat the remaining olive oil in a large skillet over high heat. Cook the cheese for 2 minutes on each side or until golden.
5. Serve the salad with the warm halloumi cheese, drizzled with the remaining balsamic vinegar.

TIP

If halloumi cheese isn't available, you can replace it with crumbled goat cheese or feta cheese, but those should not be heated up.

Green barley salad

VEGETARIAN | PREP + COOK TIME **30 MINUTES** | SERVES **6**

When in season, buy fresh fava beans in the pod. You'll need to remove the outer shell; once you blanche the favas—which helps retain their bright green color—pop the beans from their leathery gray overcoats while they're still warm. Labneh is a strained type of yogurt cheese. If you can't find it, for this recipe you may substitute your favorite kind of feta cheese.

1 cup pearl barley
1 cup frozen peas
1 cup frozen fava beans (see tips)
½ lb (150g) green beans, trimmed, halved lengthwise
1 medium cucumber, halved lengthwise, thinly sliced
6 leaves romaine lettuce, trimmed, torn
2 spring onions, thinly sliced
½ cup fresh mint leaves
2 tbsp olive oil
1 tbsp lemon juice
1½ cups (370g) labneh in olive oil, drained
salt and freshly ground black pepper

1. Place the pearl barley and 3 cups water in a medium saucepan, bring to a boil; reduce heat to low. Cook, covered, for 35 minutes or until tender. Drain; rinse under cold water until cool.
2. Meanwhile, cook the peas, fava beans, and green beans in a large saucepan of boiling water for 3 minutes or until just tender; drain. Place under cold running water to stop the cooking; drain well. Remove the gray skins from the fava beans if necessary.
3. Transfer the barley and pea mixture to a large bowl; add the cucumber, romaine lettuce, green onion, and mint. Drizzle with combined olive oil and lemon juice; toss gently to combine.
4. Top the salad with labneh cheese and season with salt and pepper to taste.

TIP

You can often find fresh fava beans at the farmers market or the organic grocery store in the spring and summer. If you use fresh, 1lb (450g) should yield about 1 cup of beans out of the pod.

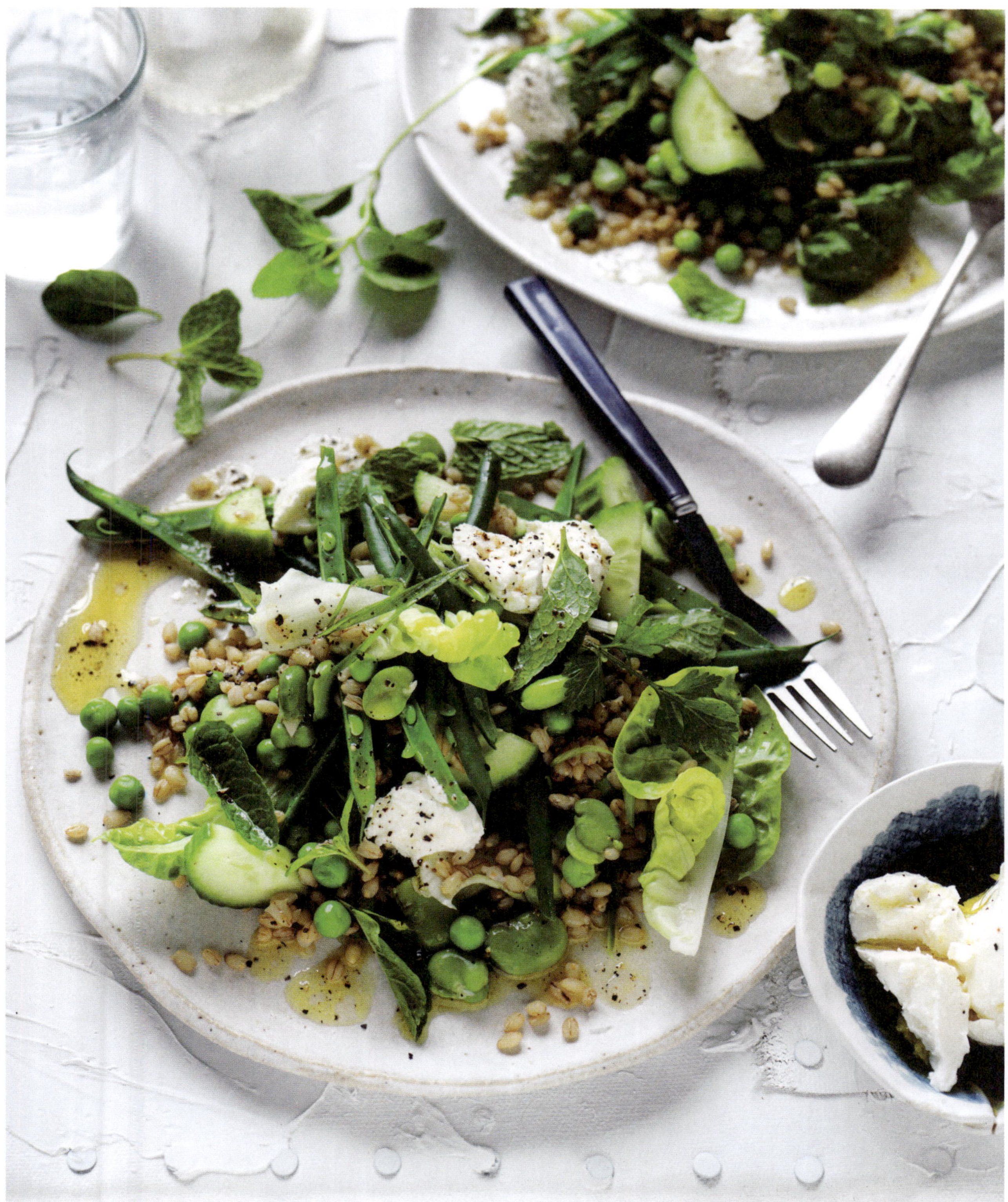

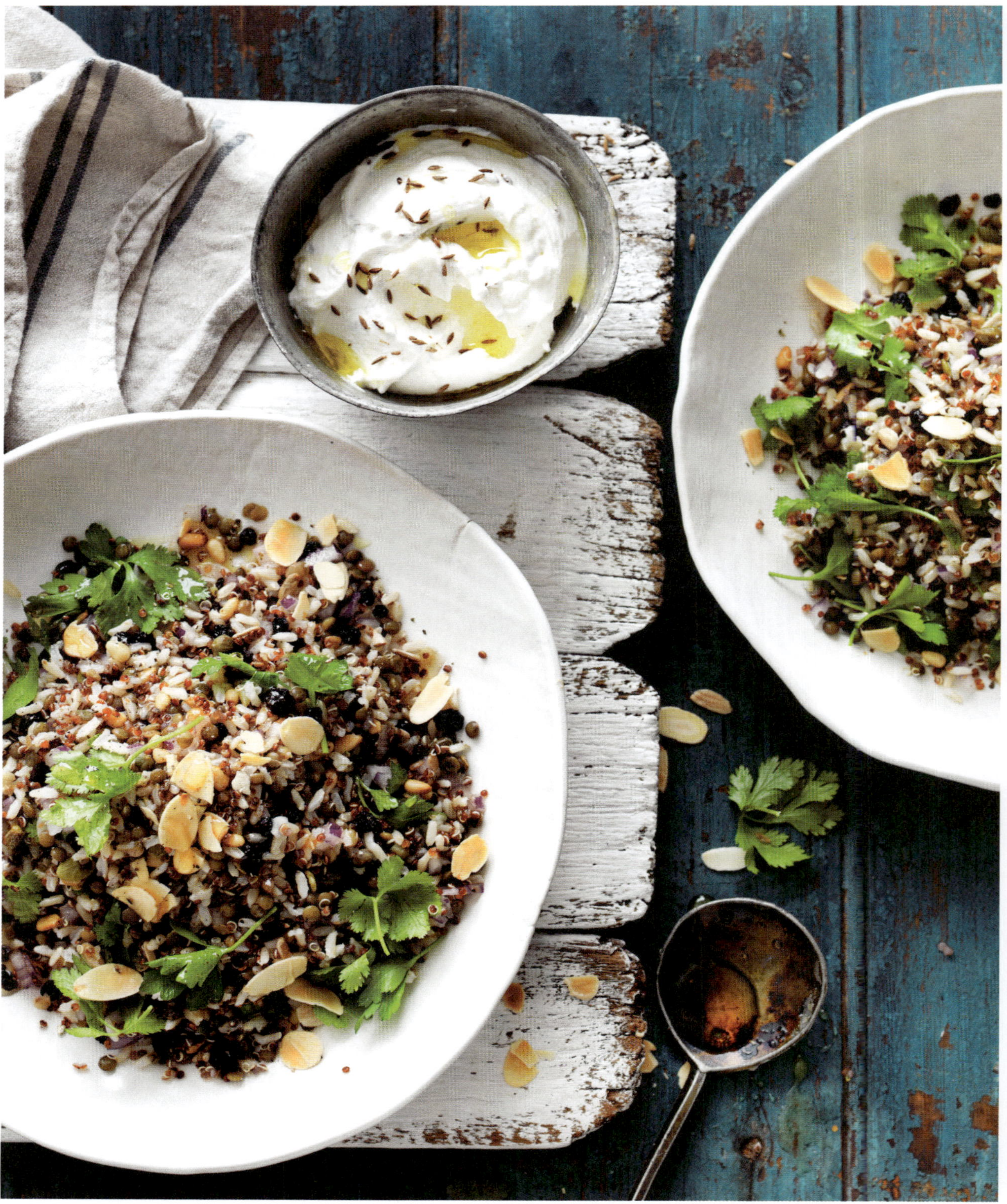

Mediterranean grain salad with honey-cumin yogurt

VEGETARIAN | PREP + COOK TIME **45 MINUTES** | SERVES **6**

Whole grains, such as the brown rice and quinoa in this recipe, are great plant sources of protein and fiber, as well as a host of vitamins, minerals, and phytochemicals that improve your health. Seeds and nuts are also packed with vitamins and minerals, as well as omega-3 fats.

3/4 cup brown rice
1/2 cup French-style green lentils, rinsed
1/2 cup red quinoa
1 small red onion, finely chopped
2 tbsp pumpkin seeds, toasted
2 tbsp sunflower seeds, toasted
2 tbsp pine nuts, toasted
2 tbsp nonpareil capers
1/2 cup dried currants
1 cup fresh Italian parsley leaves
1 cup fresh cilantro leaves
1/4 cup lemon juice
1/3 cup olive oil
1 tsp cumin seeds, toasted
1 cup Greek yogurt
1 1/2 tbsp honey
1/2 cup sliced almonds, toasted

1. Preheat the oven to 350°F (180°C). Place the seeds, pine nuts, and sliced almonds on a baking sheet, putting the cumin seeds and sliced almonds on small pieces of foil to keep them separate. Toast them for 8 minutes, stirring halfway through cooking time.
2. Meanwhile, cook the rice and lentils in separate large saucepans of boiling water for 25 minutes or until tender; drain, rinse well.
3. Place the quinoa in a small saucepan with 1 cup water, bring to a boil. Reduce heat to low; cook, covered, for 10 minutes or until tender. Drain.
4. Combine the cumin seeds and yogurt in a small bowl; drizzle with honey.
5. Place the rice, lentils, and quinoa in a large bowl. Add the onion, toasted seeds, pine nuts, capers, currants, herbs, lemon juice, and olive oil; stir until well combined. Season with salt and pepper.
6. Divide the salad among six plates; top with spoonfuls of yogurt. Sprinkle with almonds.

Spicy squash and cauliflower with rice and yogurt dressing

VEGETARIAN | PREP + COOK TIME **45 MINUTES** | SERVES **4**

Greek yogurt has been strained to remove its whey (the liquid that remains in the cheese-making process), resulting in a more sour taste and creamier texture than its more mellow counterpart. Rich in calcium, good fats, and the probiotics that are essential for good gut health, Greek yogurt is a great addition to your diet.

2lb (900g) kabocha squash, seeds removed, cut into thin wedges (see tip)

1 medium head cauliflower (about 2lb [900g]), trimmed, cut into florets

2½ tbsp olive oil, divided

2 tsp ground coriander

2 tsp ground cumin

½ tsp ground cinnamon

salt and freshly ground back pepper

½ cup brown rice

2 tsp lemon juice

1 tbsp pumpkin seeds

1 tsp finely grated lemon zest

yogurt dressing

1 cup Greek yogurt

2 tbsp fresh coriander, roughly chopped

1 tsp finely grated lemon zest

1 tbsp lemon juice

TIPS

- Instead of kabocha squash, you can use an equivalent amount of acorn squash or peeled butternut squash.
- Sprinkle with micro herbs before serving, if you like.

1. Preheat oven to 400°F (200°C). Line a large baking sheet with parchment paper.
2. Combine the squash, cauliflower, 1 tbsp of the olive oil, and the spices on a large baking sheet until the vegetables are well coated; spread evenly in a single layer. Season with salt and pepper. Roast for 30 minutes or until the vegetables are tender.
3. Meanwhile, place the rice and 8 cups water in a medium saucepan; bring to a boil. Boil for 25 minutes or until the rice is tender. Drain well; transfer to a bowl. Add the remaining olive oil and the lemon juice; stir to combine.
4. Make the yogurt dressing. Combine the ingredients in a medium bowl; season with salt and pepper to taste.
5. Spoon the rice onto a large platter or among four plates; top evenly with the roasted vegetables. Spoon on a little of the dressing, sprinkle with the pumpkin seeds and lemon rind; serve with the remaining dressing.

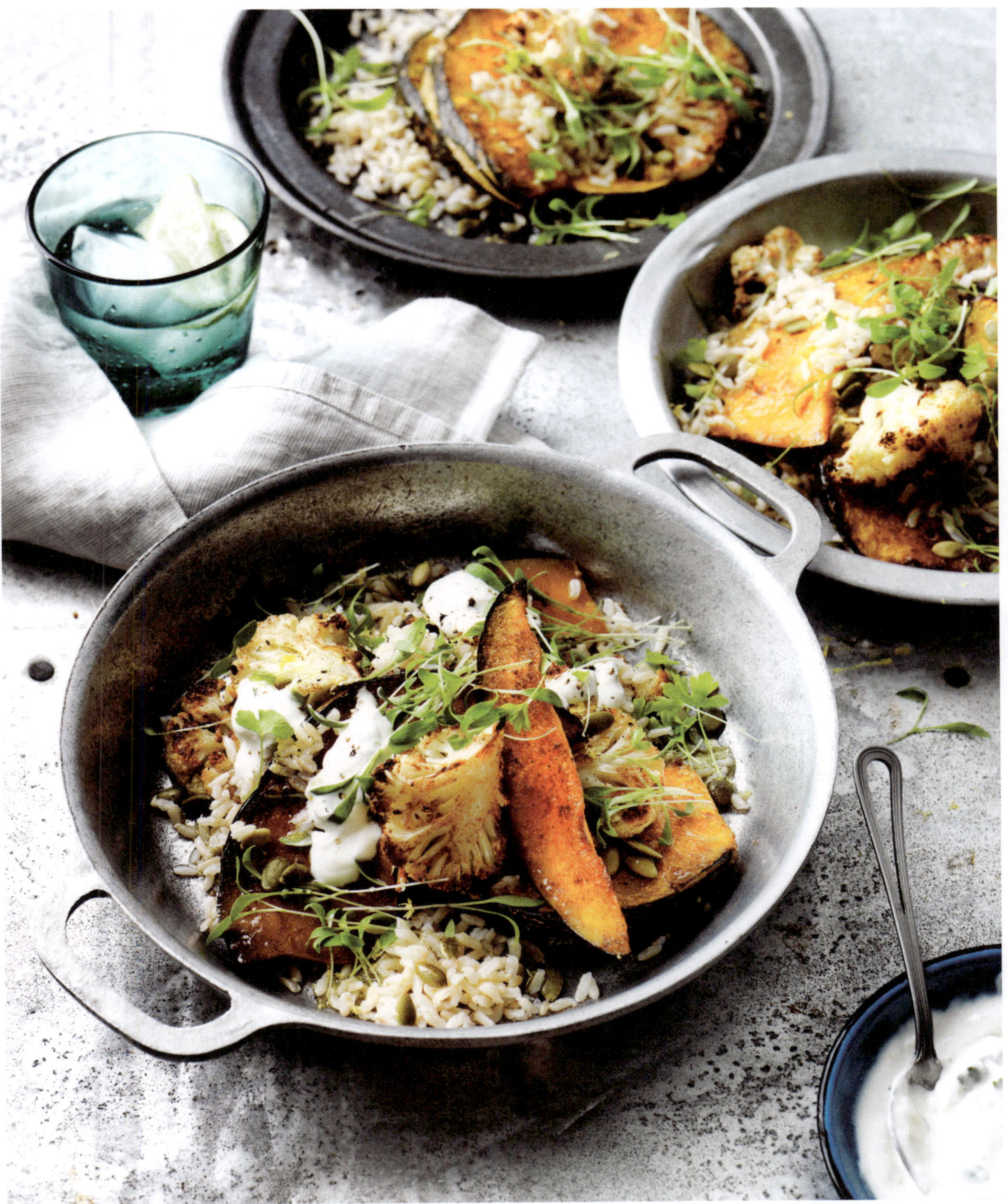

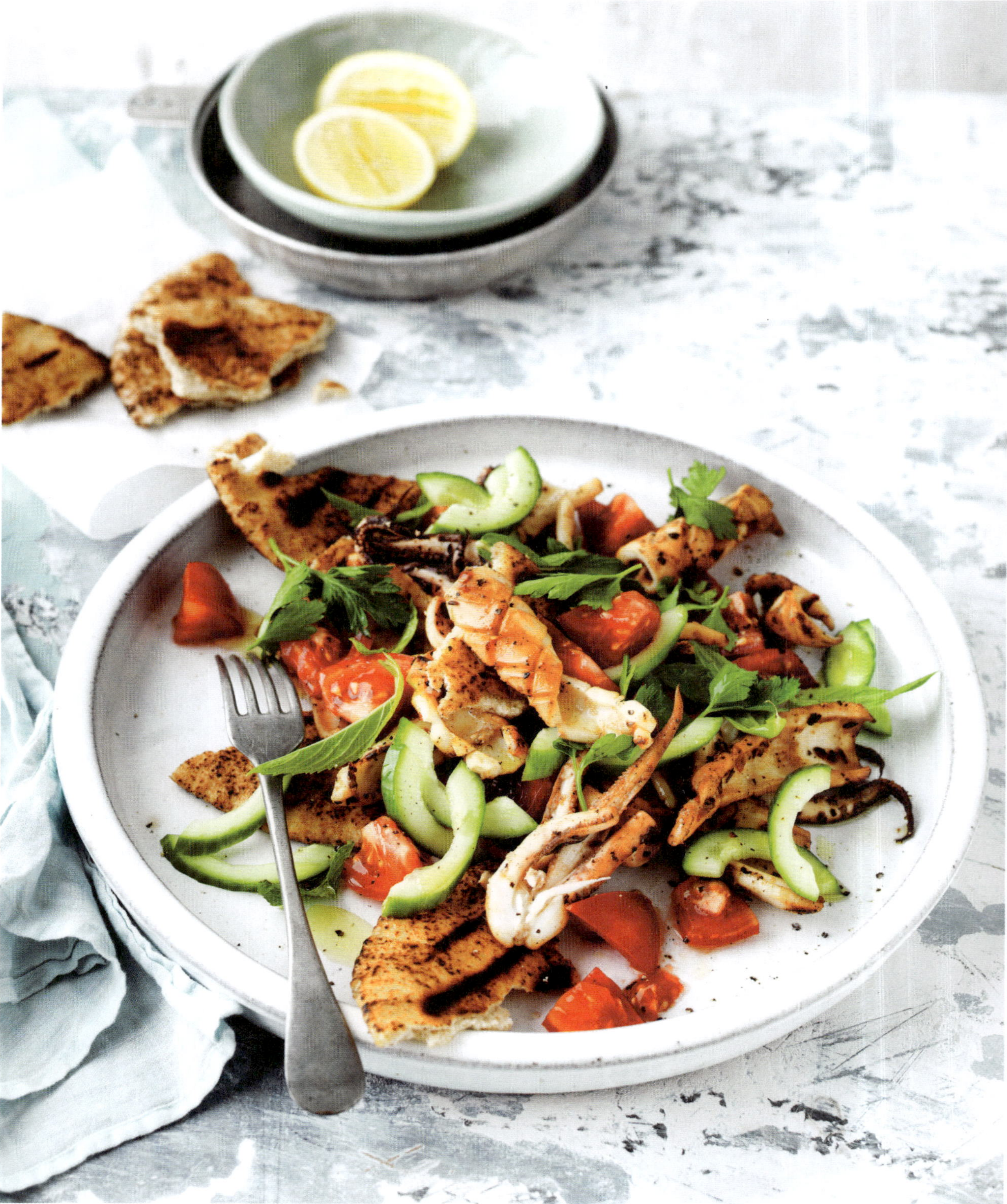

Grilled calamari fattoush salad

PESCATARIAN | PREP + COOK TIME **50 MINUTES + REFRIGERATION** | SERVES **4**

Created as a way of using day-old pita, a Lebanese fattoush salad gives new life to stale bread by frying it until crisp and combining it with fresh vegetables for texture and taste. Calamari is eaten all across the Mediterranean region. Grilled, deep fried, or stuffed, it gives flavor and color to Spanish and Italian dishes such as paella, risotto, soups, and pasta.

1½ tsp cumin seeds
1 tsp ground coriander
2 garlic cloves, crushed
½ tsp dried chile flakes
¼ cup olive oil
2 tbsp lemon juice
1½ lb (720g) calamari, cleaned (see tips)
3 medium tomatoes, roughly chopped
1½ tsp sea salt flakes
1 medium cucumber, halved lengthwise, seeded, thinly sliced
1 cup fresh mint leaves
1 cup fresh Italian parsley leaves
2 pita breads, split in half (see tips)

1. Heat a small skillet over medium heat. Cook the cumin seeds and coriander, stirring, for 2 minutes or until toasted and fragrant. Transfer to a medium bowl, add the garlic, chile, olive oil, and lemon juice; stir to combine. Reserve 2 tbsp of the spice mixture in a small bowl.
2. Cut the calamari hoods in half lengthwise. Score the inside surface of the calamari in a criss-cross pattern at ½in (1cm) intervals. Cut into 1½in (4cm) strips. Add the calamari hoods and tentacles to the spice mixture in the bowl; toss to coat. Refrigerate the calamari for 2 hours.
3. Meanwhile, combine the tomato and salt in a colander; let it stand in the sink for 10 minutes to drain. Place the tomato, cucumber, mint, and parsley in a medium bowl; toss to combine.
4. Cook the pita and calamari hoods and tentacles on a heated oiled grill or ridged grill pan until the pita are toasted and the calamari is just cooked through.
5. Break the pita into bite-sized pieces. Add the reserved spice mixture and half the pita to the tomato mixture; toss to combine. Serve the calamari with the salad and remaining pita.

TIPS

- Look for cleaned squid at your fish counter.
- If you're having difficulty splitting the pita breads open, microwave on high (100%) for 10 seconds. The steam from heating in the microwave usually makes it easier to open the bread.

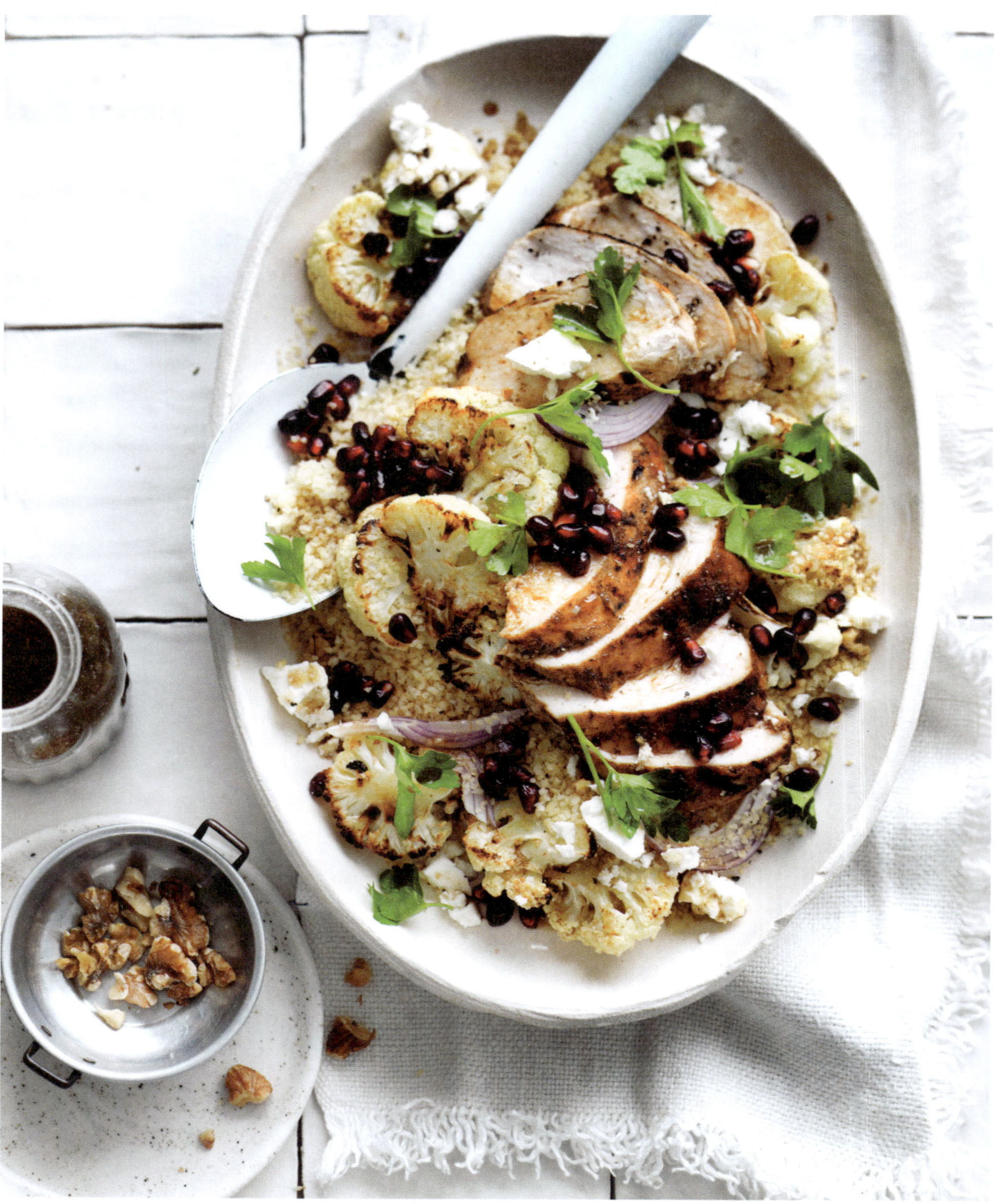

Chicken, bulgur, and pomegranate salad

PREP + COOK TIME **45 MINUTES + REFRIGERATION AND STANDING** | SERVES **6**

Pomegranates have been cultivated in the Mediterranean since ancient times; their bright red seeds, or arils, feature heavily in the region's art and literature, as well as its cuisine. Look for pomegranate molasses in delis, Middle Eastern markets, and specialty food shops.

1/4 cup olive oil, divided
1/4 cup pomegranate molasses
1 tbsp ground cumin
2 garlic cloves, crushed
4 boneless, skinless chicken breasts (about 1 1/2lb [700g])
1 1/2 cups chicken stock
1 1/2 cups bulgur
1 head cauliflower (about 2lb [1 kg])
salt and freshly ground black pepper
1 cup pomegranate seeds (see tip)
1 medium red onion, halved, thinly sliced
1 cup fresh Italian parsley leaves
1 cup coarsely chopped walnuts, roasted
1/2 cup feta cheese, crumbled

pomegranate dressing

1/4 cup olive oil
1/4 cup lemon juice
3 tsp honey
3 tsp pomegranate molasses

1 Combine 2 tbsp of the olive oil, the molasses, cumin, and garlic in a large bowl; add the chicken and turn to coat. Cover; refrigerate for 3 hours or overnight.

2 Bring the stock to a boil in a medium saucepan. Remove from the heat, add the bulgur; cover, let stand for 5 minutes.

3 Meanwhile, preheat a grill (barbecue) or ridged grill pan. Trim the cauliflower; cut into 1in (2.5cm) florets. Place on an oven tray; drizzle with the remaining olive oil, season with salt and pepper. Grill the cauliflower for 8 minutes, turning halfway through cooking time, or until tender.

4 Make the pomegranate dressing. Place the ingredients in a screw-top jar; shake well. Season with salt and pepper to taste.

5 Drain the chicken; discard the marinade. Cook the chicken on a heated oil grill (barbecue) or ridged grill pan for 4 minutes on each side or until cooked through. Let stand, covered loosely with foil, for 10 minutes. Slice thickly.

6 Spoon the bulgur onto a platter or bowl; top with the chicken, cauliflower, pomegranate seeds, onion, parsley, walnuts, and feta cheese. Drizzle with the dressing.

TIP

One pomegranate typically yields 1 cup seeds. To remove seeds, cut fruit in half crosswise; hold a half, cut-side down, in palm, over a small bowl; hit the outside firmly with a wooden spoon. Discard any white pith. Repeat with other half.

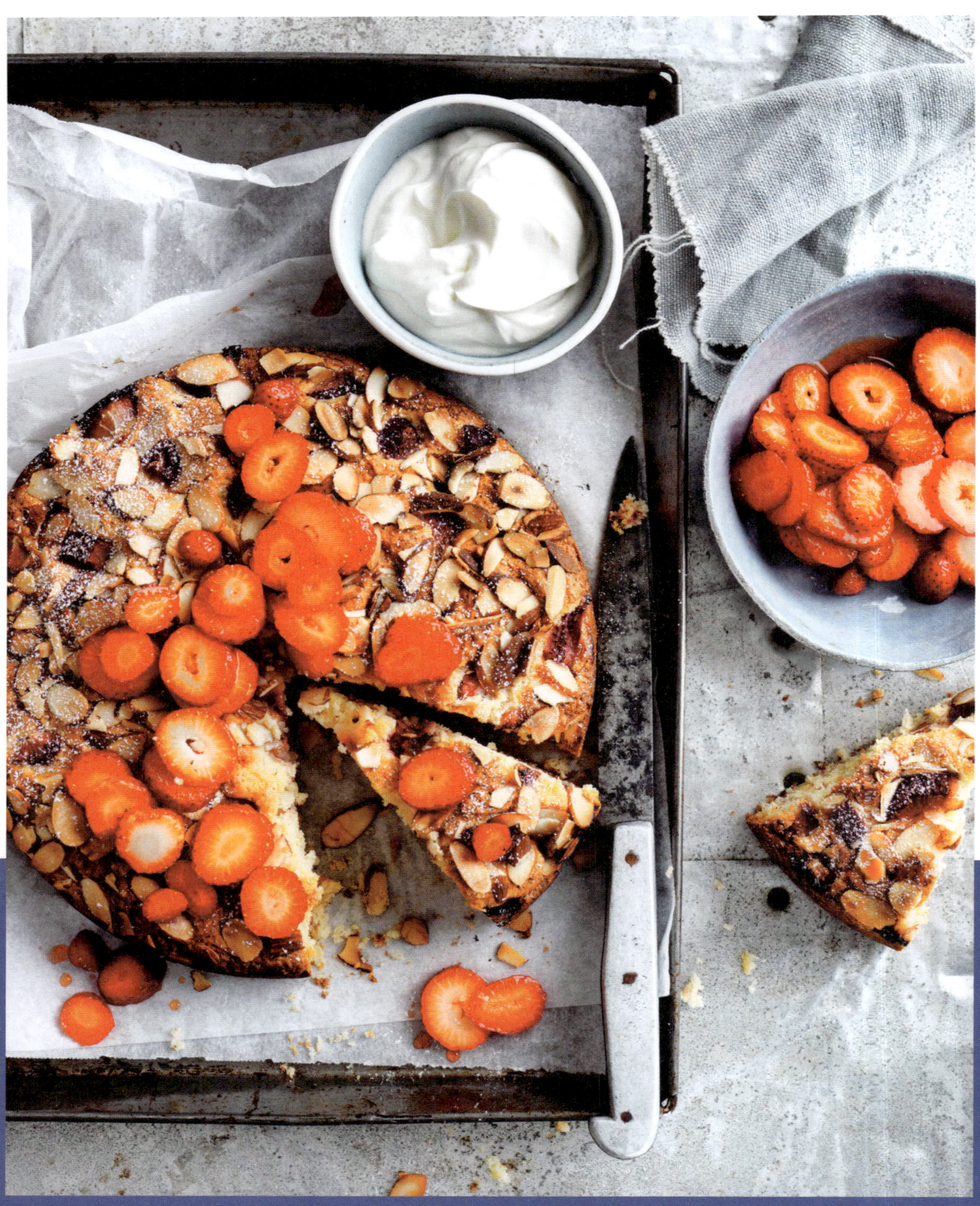

DESSERTS

Round off your meal with the sweet flavors of the Mediterranean—figs, fruit compotes, honey, cakes, and baklava all star in this mouthwatering collection of desserts.

Spiced couscous with passionfruit yogurt

PREP + COOK TIME **25 MINUTES** | SERVES **4**

Couscous consists of steamed balls of crushed durum wheat semolina; it has a similar nutritional value to pasta. Originally a North African dish, it traveled to the Mediterranean in the 17th century, and is now widely eaten in the region. For this recipe, you may swap the blueberries for strawberries or raspberries, or use a mixture of all three.

1 cup whole wheat couscous

2 tsp olive oil

1/2 tsp cinnamon

1/2 tsp nutmeg

1/4 tsp allspice

1/4 cup honey

1/2 cup walnuts, toasted, chopped

3/4 cup Greek yogurt

2 tbsp frozen or canned passion fruit purée or passionfruit concentrate, seeds removed (see tip)

2 medium oranges

1/3 cup blueberries

2 tbsp fresh mint leaves

1 Combine the couscous, olive oil, cinnamon, nutmeg, allspice, honey, and a pinch of salt with 1 cup boiling water in a medium bowl. Let stand, covered, for 5 minutes or until all the liquid is absorbed. Fluff with a fork. Stir in the walnuts.

2 Meanwhile, combine the yogurt and passionfruit in a small bowl.

3 Finely grate the zest from one orange; you will need 1 tsp. Peel the oranges, then thinly slice. Serve the spiced couscous topped with the orange slices, blueberries, passionfruit, yogurt, mint, and orange zest.

TIP

Passionfruit purée can sometimes be found in the freezer section or in cans. Bottled concentrate has water and seeds removed and works perfectly for this recipe, as does pulp.

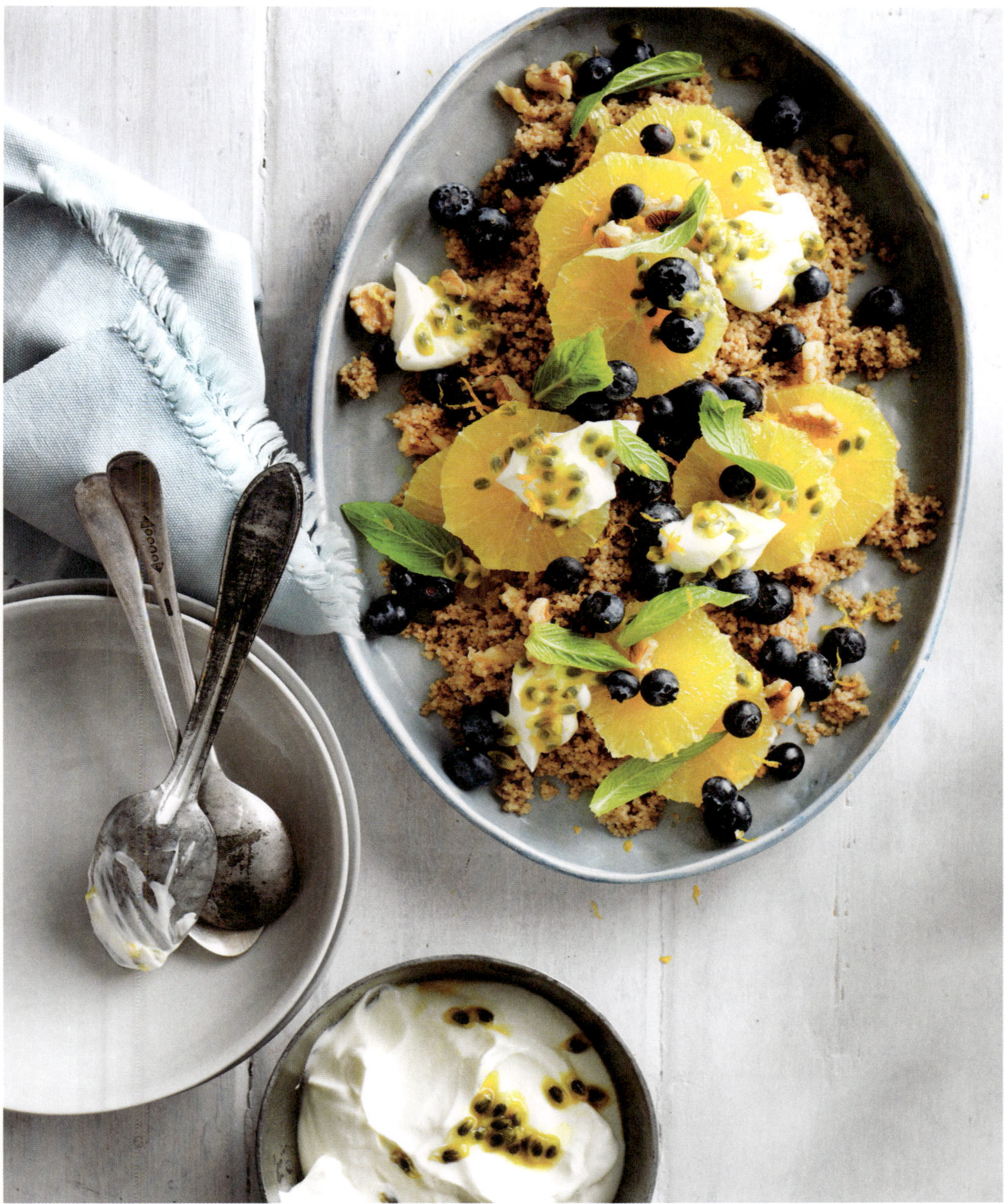

Honey and cherry barley pudding

PREP + COOK TIME **50 MINUTES** | SERVES **2**

One of the first cultivated grains in history, barley is a wonderfully versatile grain with a rich nutty flavor and packed with fiber. Here it's used in a sweet pudding, but it can also bulk out a vegetable soup or replace red meat in a hearty winter stew. Sheep's milk yogurt and fresh honeycomb can be purchased from health food stores and organic supermarkets.

$^{1}/_{2}$ cup pearl barley (see tips)
1 cup (280g) plain sheep's milk yogurt
$^{1}/_{2}$ tsp ground cinnamon
1$^{1}/_{2}$ cups frozen pitted cherries, thawed, halved, divided (see tips)
1oz (30g) fresh honeycomb, sliced
2 tbsp blanched almonds, chopped
ground cinnamon, extra, to serve

1 Place the barley and 1$^{1}/_{2}$ cups water in a small saucepan, bring to a boil. Reduce heat to low; cook, covered, for 35 minutes or until tender. Drain. Rinse under cold water until cool; drain well.

2 In a large bowl, combine the cooked barley, yogurt, cinnamon, and $^{2}/_{3}$ cup of the cherries. To serve, divide the mixture between two bowls. Top with the remaining cherries, the honeycomb, and the almonds; dust with the extra ground cinnamon.

TIPS

- You could also try this with cooked quinoa instead of pearl barley.
- Frozen raspberries can be used instead of cherries.
- Use fresh pitted cherries when in season.

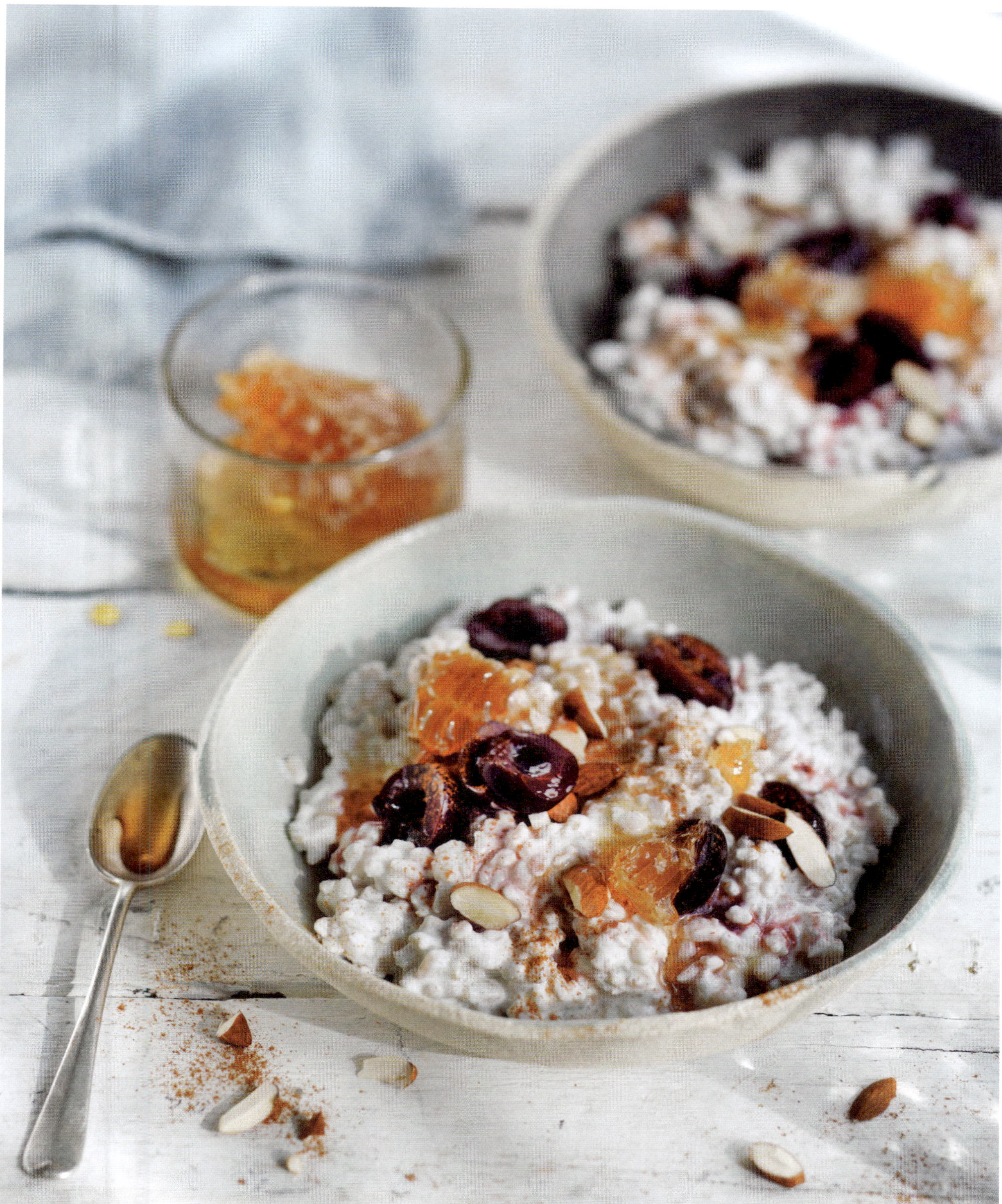

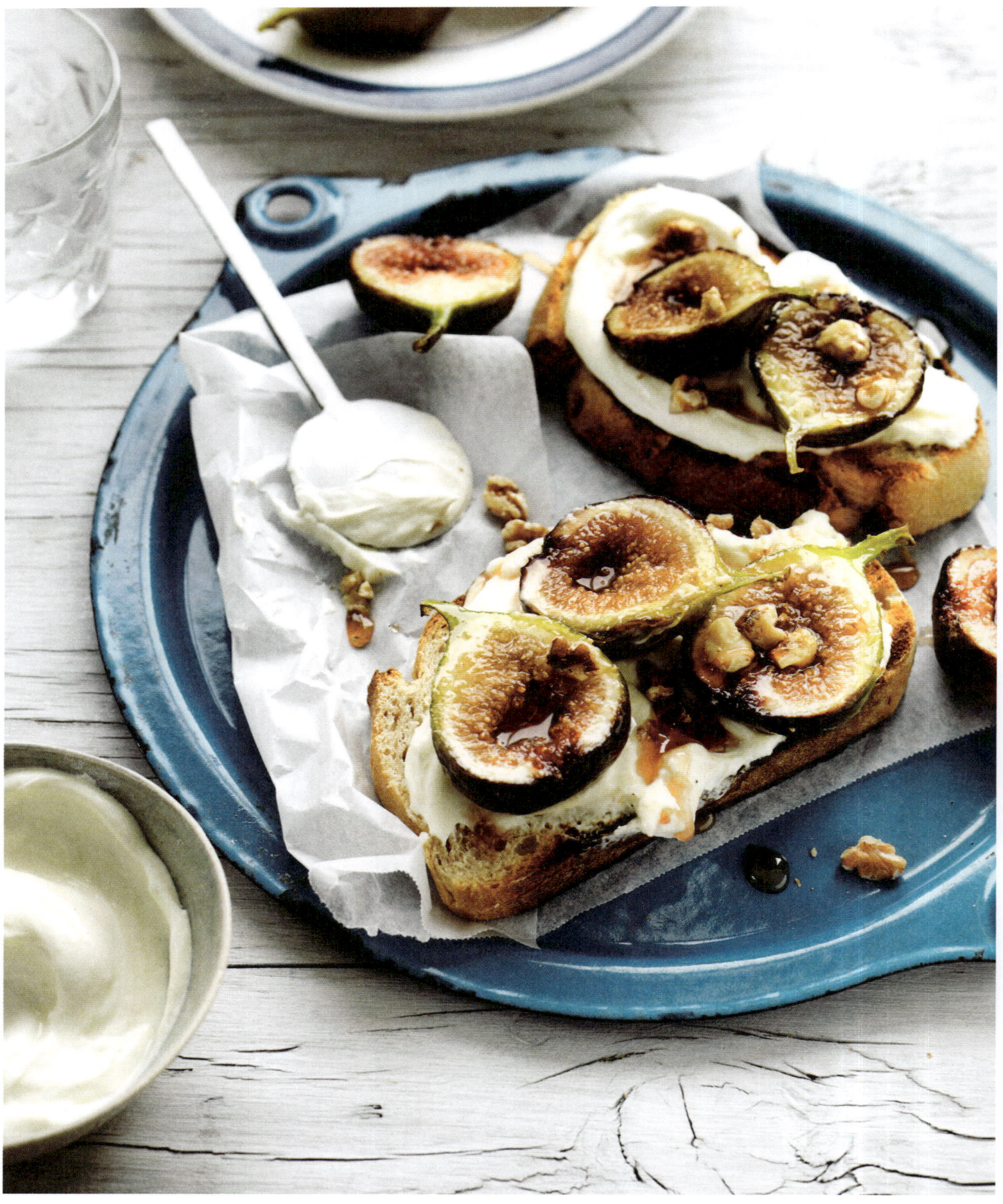

Sweet fig bruschetta

PREP + COOK TIME **10 MINUTES** | SERVES **4**

Figs are one of the most recognizable Mediterranean fruits, featuring heavily in the art and myths of the region. In fact, figs are thought to be the first fruit to be cultivated by humans for food, and they were widely consumed in ancient Greece and Rome. Try to use local honey for this recipe, rather than commercial honey, which has been highly refined.

6 fresh figs, halved
1/3 cup honey
1 tbsp powdered sugar
1/3 cup mascarpone cheese
2/3 cup Greek yogurt
4 slices sourdough bread, 1/2in (1cm) thick, toasted
2 tbsp walnuts, roughly chopped (see tip)

1 Heat a large nonstick pan over medium-high heat. Drizzle the cut sides of the figs with honey. Cook the figs, cut-side down, for 2 minutes or until glazed and warmed through. Add 2 tbsp cold water to the pan; remove from heat.

2 Meanwhile, whisk the sifted powdered sugar, mascarpone cheese, and yogurt in a small bowl until combined.

3 Spread the toast evenly with the mascarpone cheese mixture; top with the figs and walnuts. Before serving, drizzle with the cooking juices.

TIP

You can use chopped pistachios or sliced almonds instead of walnuts, if you like.

Whole orange semolina cake with rosemary syrup

PREP + COOK TIME **2 HOURS 40 MINUTES + STANDING** | SERVES **12**

Semolina is a coarsely ground flour milled from the hardest part (endosperm) of the durum wheat grain. It's commonly used in making gnocchi, pasta, and couscous. Although it's not gluten-free, it is high in potassium, digests more slowly than white flour, and is fiber-rich. Here it imparts a rich, nutty flavor to the cake, kept extra moist with the aromatic syrup.

2 large oranges
1 tsp baking powder
6 eggs
1 cup sugar
1 cup fine semolina
1¼ cups almond meal
1½ tsp finely chopped fresh rosemary

rosemary syrup
2 large oranges
½ cup sugar
1½ tbsp lemon juice
2 tbsp orange-flavored liqueur
3 sprigs fresh rosemary

1 Place the unpeeled oranges in a medium saucepan, cover with cold water; bring to a boil. Cook, covered, for 1½ hours or until the oranges are tender; drain. Let cool.

2 Preheat oven to 350°F (180°C). Grease a 9in (23cm) springform pan; cut out a 9in (23cm) circle of parchment paper; line bottom of pan with it.

3 Trim and discard the ends of the cooked oranges. Halve; discard the seeds. In the bowl of a food processor, add the orange halves (with rind) and baking powder. Pulse until the mixture is pulpy. Transfer to a large bowl.

4 In a large mixing bowl, cream the sugar and eggs for 5 minutes until thick and light colored. Stir in the orange mixture. Fold in the semolina, almond meal, and rosemary. Spread the mixture into the lined pan.

5 Bake the cake for 1 hour or until a toothpick inserted into the center comes out clean; cover loosely with foil halfway during baking if it's getting too brown. Leave cake to cool in the pan for 5 minutes. Unclasp the springform pan and remove. Transfer the cake (including the parchment) onto a cake plate to serve.

6 Meanwhile, to make the rosemary syrup, zest one orange in long thin strips. For the second orange, use the vegetable peeler to remove one long continuous strip of rind, avoiding any of the white pith. Place the sugar, lemon juice, and ½ cup water in a small saucepan over low heat; stir, without boiling, until the sugar dissolves. Add the thin strips and long strip of orange rind, bring to a boil; boil for 5 minutes or until the syrup thickens. Remove from the heat; stir in the liqueur and rosemary.

7 Spoon the hot syrup and candied orange rind strips over the warm cake. Serve the cake warm or at room temperature.

TIP

If you don't have a zester, simply peel the rind into wide strips with a vegetable peeler.

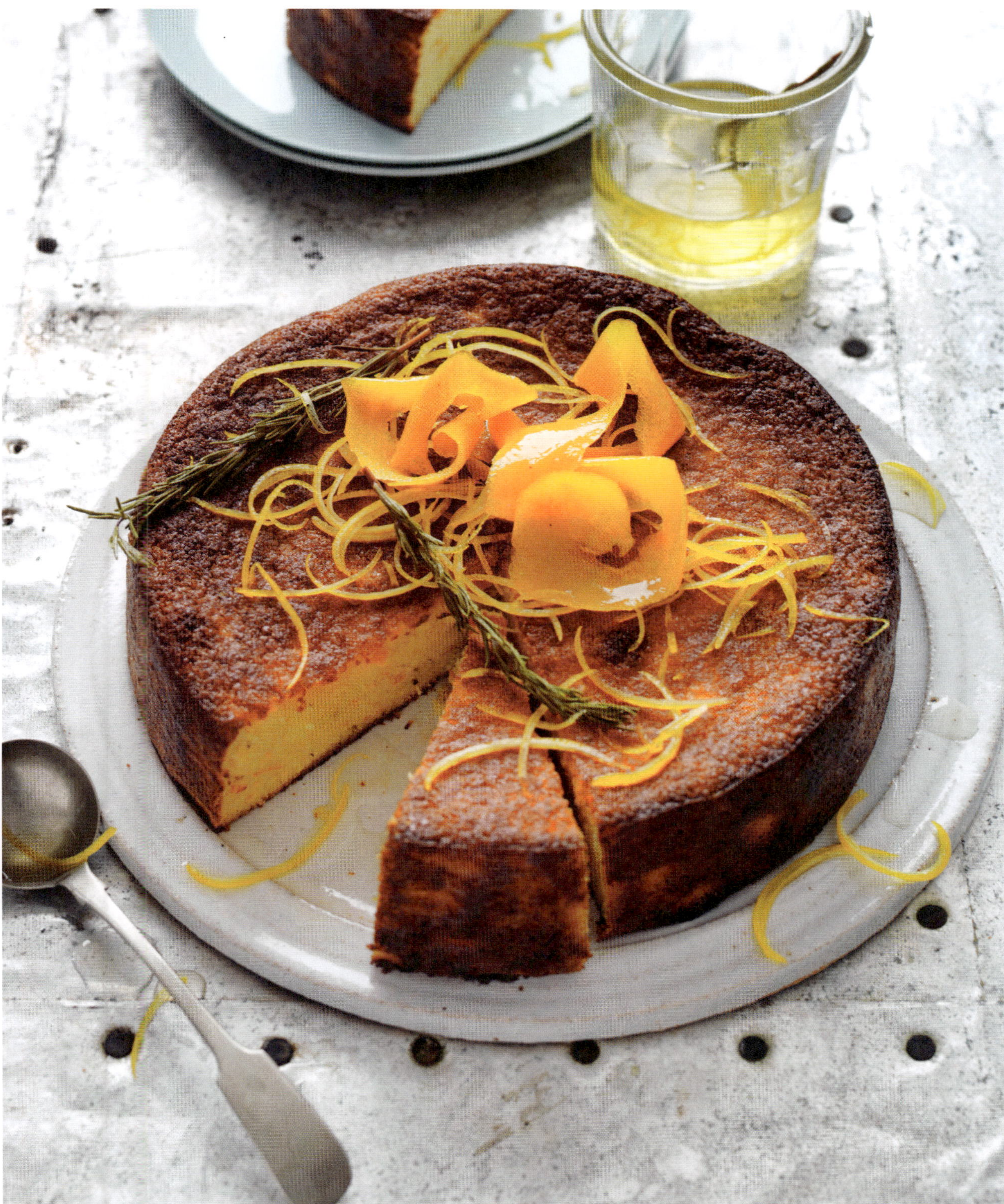

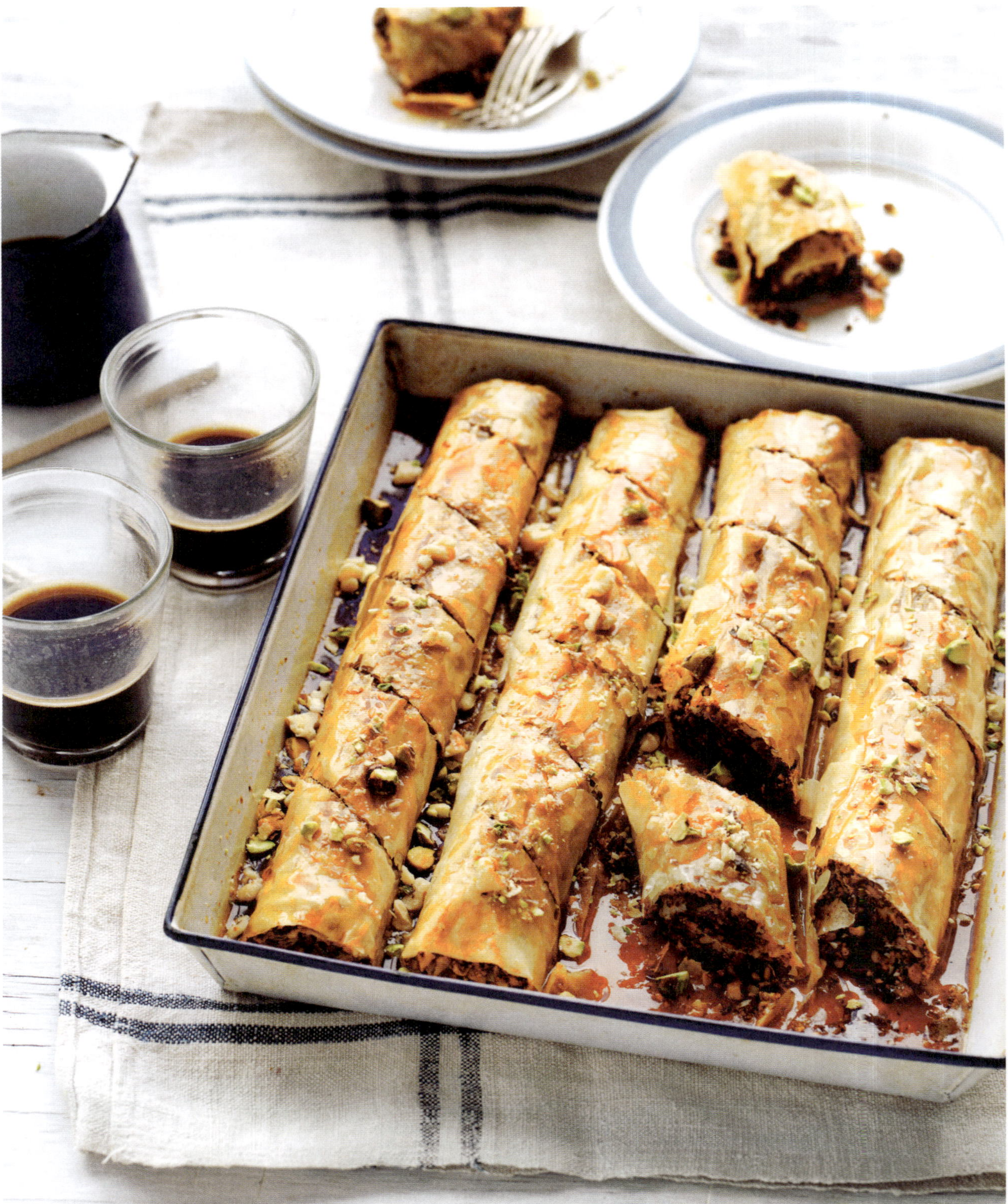

Pistachio, walnut, and chocolate baklava

PREP + COOK TIME **1 HOUR 10 MINUTES + STANDING** | MAKES **36**

Baklava is probably the most recognizable of all sweet Greek pastries, with its origins dating back to the Ottoman Empire. It's a rich, sticky dessert made of layers of phyllo pastry filled with chopped nuts and held together with either a sugar syrup or honey. We've added dark chocolate to our version of baklava, to up the decadent level of this sweet treat.

8 sheets phyllo dough, 14 x 18in (36 x 46cm), thawed
8 tbsp unsalted butter, melted
2 tbsp finely chopped pistachios

pistachio and walnut filling

1½ cups pistachios
2 cups walnuts
1½ cups semi-sweet chocolate chips
⅓ cup sugar
2 tsp ground cinnamon
1½ tbsp finely grated orange zest

honey syrup

1 medium orange
1½ cups sugar
½ cup honey
⅓ cup orange juice

TIP

Serve with Greek yogurt, sprinkled with finely grated or thinly sliced orange rind, if you like.

1. Preheat oven to 350°F (180°C). Line a large large baking sheet with parchment paper. Butter a 9 x 9in (23cm) ovenproof casserole.
2. To make the pistachio and walnut filling, spread the pistachios and walnuts on the baking sheet. Toast for 5 minutes until the nuts begin to turn golden brown, stirring once to cook evenly. Let cool. In the bowl of a food processor, add the nuts, the chocolate chips, sugar, cinnamon, and orange zest. Pulse until finely chopped.
3. Increase the oven to 375°F(190°C). On a dry surface or parchment paper sheet, layer four pastry sheets, brushing each with the butter. Keep the remaining sheets covered with a clean, damp kitchen towel to prevent drying. Spread a quarter of the filling over the pastry sheets, leaving a 1in (2.5cm) border along both long sides. Starting on a long side, roll the pastry up to form a log. Cut the log in half. Place both halves in the buttered dish. Brush with butter. Repeat with the remaining pastry sheets, filling, and butter.
4. Bake the baklava for 20 minutes or until golden.
5. Meanwhile, make the honey syrup. Remove zest from the orange in long thin strips with a zester. Juice the orange for ⅓ cup of orange juice. Stir the orange zest strips, sugar, honey, and 1½ cups water in a small saucepan, over medium heat, without boiling, until the sugar dissolves. Bring to a simmer; cook for 10 minutes or until slightly thickened. Stir in the orange juice.
6. Cool the baklava for 5 minutes, then cut each log on the diagonal into ¾in (2cm) wide pieces. Pour the hot syrup over the baklava; let stand for 3 hours or until the syrup is absorbed. Serve topped with chopped pistachios.

Raspberry ricotta cheesecake

PREP + COOK TIME **1 HOUR 30 MINUTES + REFRIGERATION AND COOLING** | SERVES **8**

Ricotta cheese makes for a lighter dessert than the traditional cheesecake made with cream cheese. Amaretti are Italian cookies made from almonds; legend has it they were created to welcome a visiting cardinal to the town of Saronno. The recipe for the cookies was supposedly kept a family secret over many generations.

2 cups amaretti cookies(see tip)
2 tbsp sugar
5 tbsp unsalted butter, melted
1 cup raspberries
2 tbsp powdered sugar
1 cup raspberries, extra
2 tsp powdered sugar, extra

raspberry ricotta cheese filling
2 cups cream cheese
1¼ cup ricotta cheese
1 cup sugar
⅓ cup milk
3 eggs
1 cup raspberries

1 Grease an 8in (20cm) springform pan.

2 In a food processor, add the cookies and the sugar. Pulse until fine crumbs form. With the processor running, gradually add the butter until well combined. Press the cookie mixture over the bottom of the pan, using the back of a spoon to smooth the mixture and press it tightly in place. Place the pan on a baking sheet; refrigerate for 30 minutes.

3 Preheat oven to 300°F (150°C).

4 To make the raspberry ricotta cheese filling, in a large bowl, combine the cheeses, sugar, and milk until smooth. Add the eggs and mix until combined. Fold in the raspberries. Pour the filling into the prepared springform pan.

5 Bake for 50 minutes or until the cheesecake is cooked around the edge and slightly wobbly in the middle. Turn oven off; let the cheesecake cool in the oven for 1 hour with the door ajar. (The top of the cheesecake may crack slightly while cooling.) Refrigerate for 4 hours or overnight, until firm.

6 In a food processor or blender, add the raspberries, powdered sugar, and water; purée. Strain through a sieve into a small bowl. Spread some purée over the cheesecake, top with extra raspberries; dust with extra powdered sugar. Serve with the remaining purée.

TIPS

- If you can't find amaretti cookies, substitute 2 cups crushed graham crackers, pulsing them with 1 tsp almond extract in a food processor.
- Depending on the design of the springform pan, clip the base in upside down so the base is level; this makes it easier to remove the cheesecake.

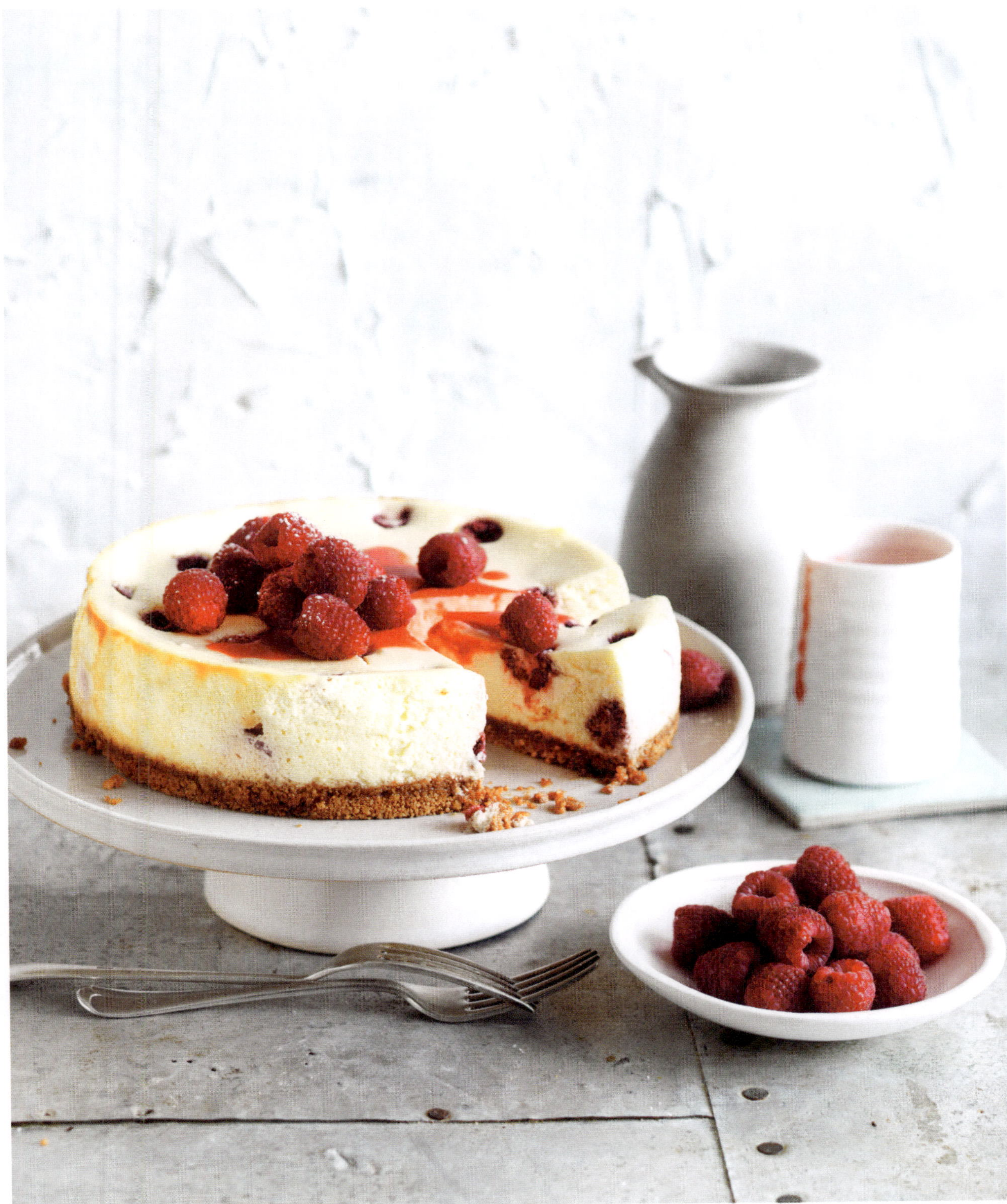

Fruit compote

Fruit compote is great paired with yogurt or muesli, or try stirring it into your oatmeal or hot cereal to liven up your breakfast. To turn a compote into a dessert, add a crumble topping and bake, or serve with ice cream and waffles.

Pear, cardamom, and ginger

VEGAN | PREP + COOK TIME **45 MINUTES** | SERVES **4**

Place 4 peeled, cored, and thickly sliced Bartlett pears in a medium saucepan with 1 cup water, 2 tsp of freshly grated ginger, 6 bruised cardamom pods, 1 cinnamon stick, and 1 tbsp of lemon juice; bring to a boil. Reduce heat; simmer, partially covered, for 25 minutes, stirring occasionally, or until the liquid has reduced slightly and the pears are tender. Serve warm or chilled.

Vanilla-roasted nectarines and peaches

VEGAN | PREP TIME **35 MINUTES** | SERVES **4**

Preheat oven to 425°F (220°C). Butter a 9 x 9in (23 x 23cm) heatproof casserole. Halve and remove the pits from 3 medium yellow nectarines and 3 medium yellow peaches; place in the dish. Split a vanilla bean lengthwise; scrape seeds from the halves, using the tip of a knife. Add the vanilla bean and seeds to the dish with 2 tbsp of pure maple syrup, 2 x 1½in (4cm) strips of lemon zest, 1 tbsp of lemon juice, and a pinch of sea salt flakes; turn the fruit to coat it. Arrange the fruit in a single layer, cut-side up. Bake the fruit for 20 minutes or until the fruit is tender but still holds its shape. Serve warm or chilled.

Apple, rhubarb, and goji

VEGAN | PREP TIME **25 MINUTES** | SERVES **4**

Place ½ cup fresh orange juice and 2 tbsp of maple syrup in a medium saucepan over low heat; cook, stirring, until the syrup melts. Add 2 large coarsely chopped Pink Lady apples, a 1½in (4cm) wide strip of orange zest, and the seeds scraped from half a vanilla bean plus its pod; simmer, covered, for 5 minutes. Add 1 bunch trimmed, coarsely chopped rhubarb and 2 tbsp of goji berries; simmer gently, covered, for 10 minutes or until the fruit is tender and still holding its shape. Serve warm or chilled.

Plum, raspberry, and rosemary

VEGAN | PREP TIME **25 MINUTES** | SERVES **4**

Halve and remove the pits from 5 red or black plums; cut each half into thirds. Place the plums in a large saucepan with ¼ cup water, 1 tbsp of lemon juice, 1 cinnamon stick, and 2 sprigs fresh rosemary; bring to a boil. Reduce heat; simmer, covered, for 5 minutes. Uncover; simmer for 5 more minutes or until the plums are just tender. Stir in ½ cup raspberries and 2 tsp of monk fruit sugar until the monk fruit sugar dissolves. Remove from the heat.

CLOCKWISE from top left

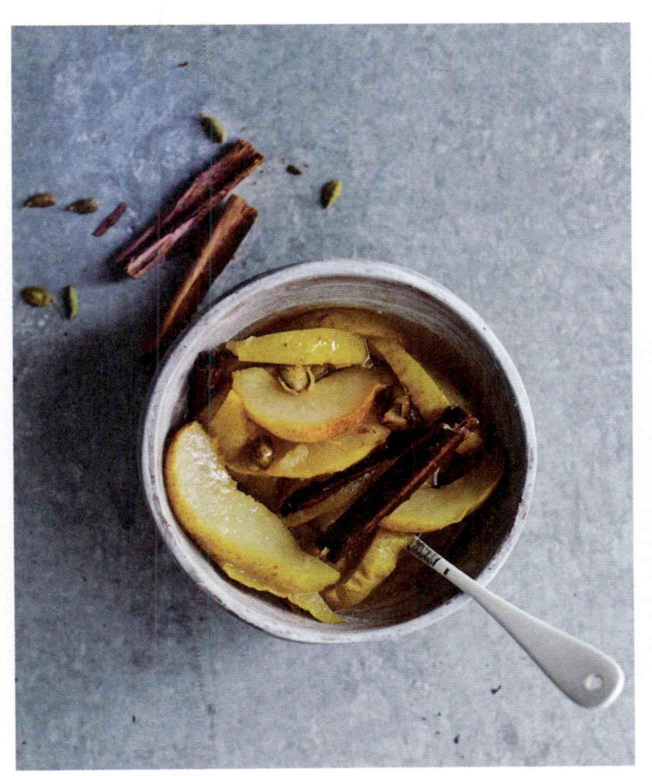
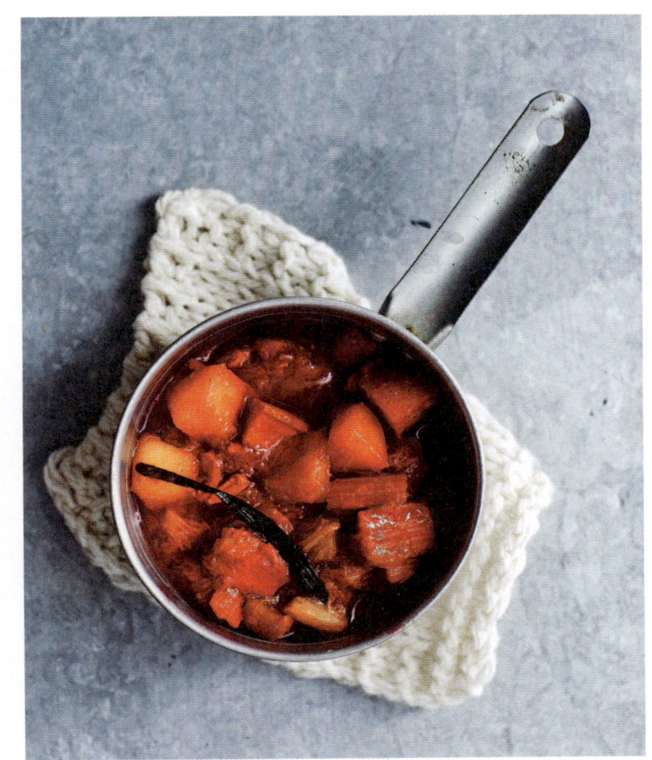
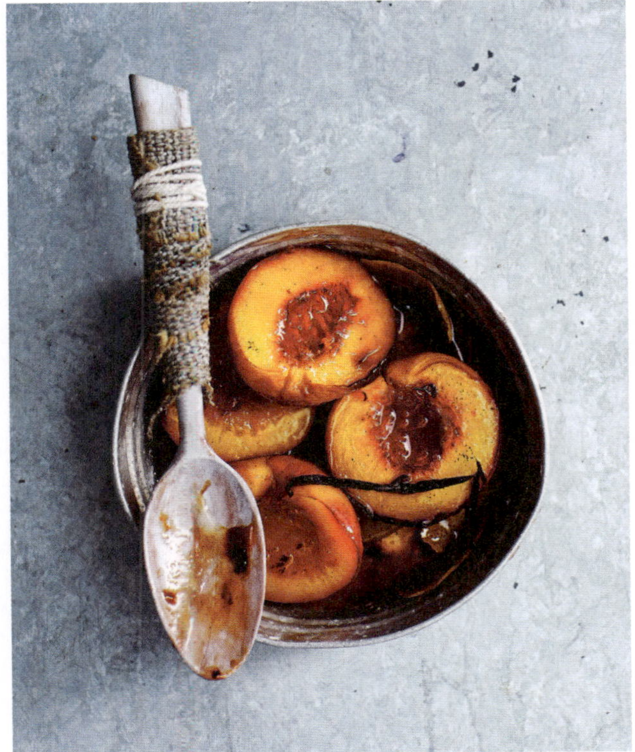
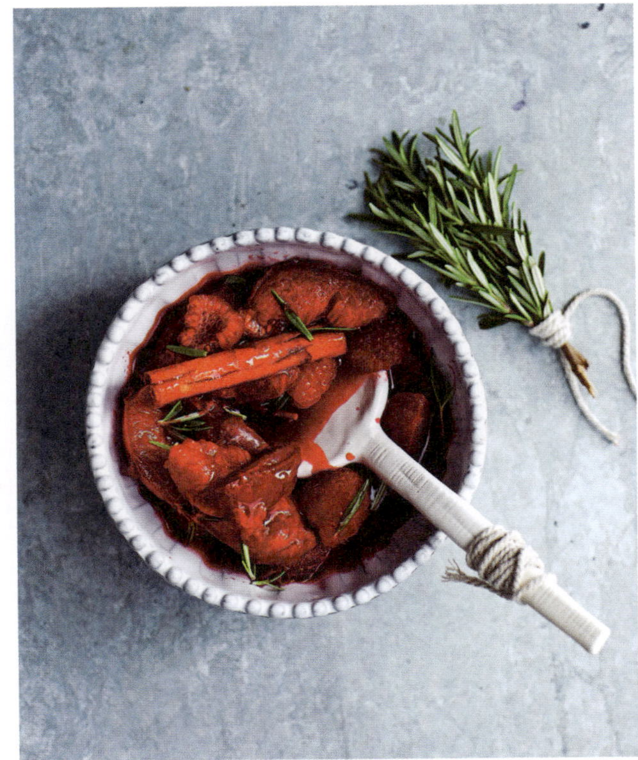

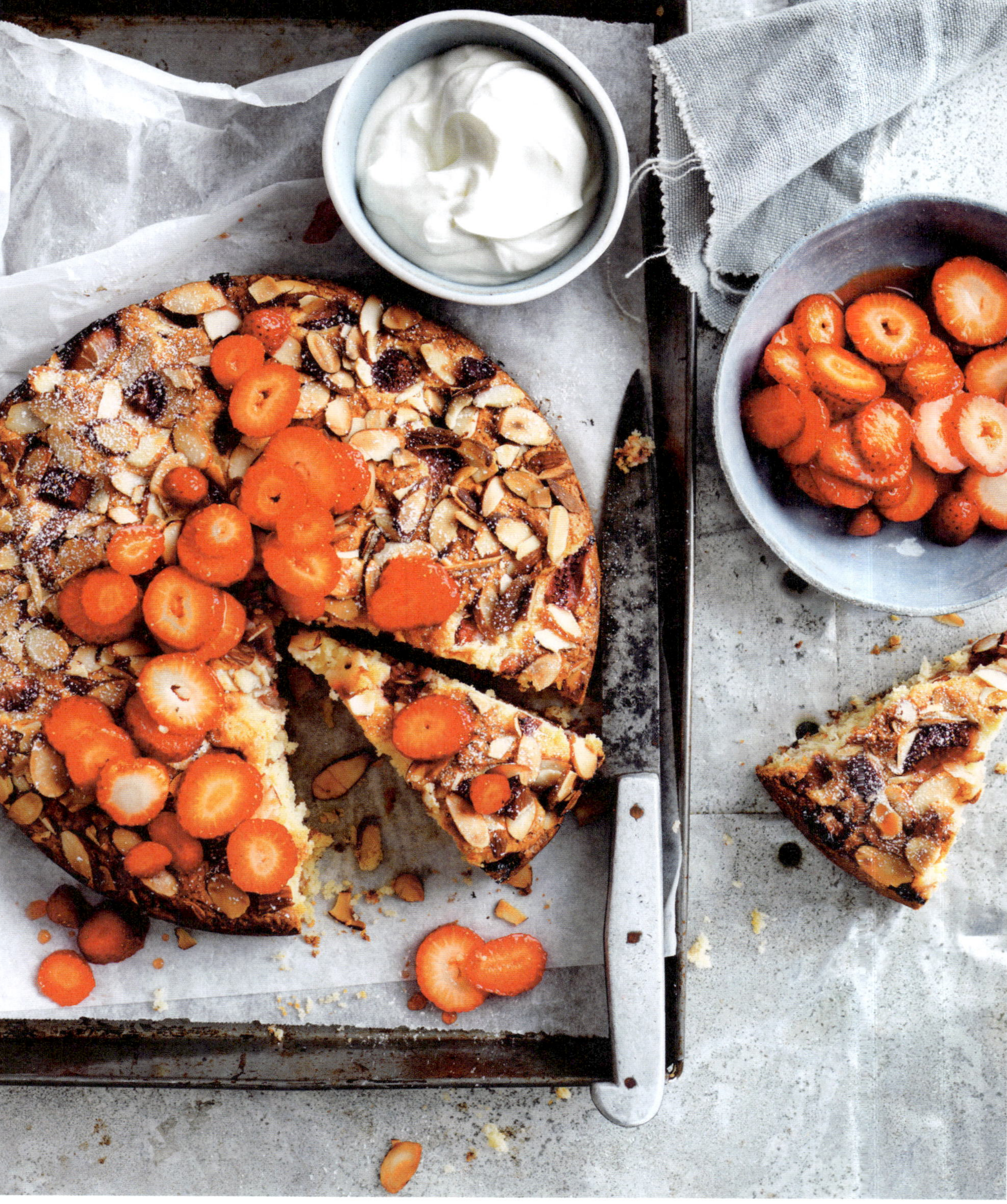

Melt 'n' mix strawberry yogurt cake

PREP + COOK TIME **1 HOUR 15 MINUTES + COOLING** | SERVES **8**

Mediterranean desserts sometimes have the reputation of being overly fussy—though meals are often concluded simply with fresh fruits, some sharp cheese, and a nighttime tipple. Here we have a moist and nutty cake that requires no more than one bowl to prepare, so there's no excuse not to indulge in a freshly baked cake for dessert.

2½ cups all-purpose flour
3 tsp baking powder
1¼ tsp baking soda
1 tsp salt
2 cups strawberries, coarsely chopped
1 cup sugar
1 tsp vanilla extract
2 eggs, lightly beaten
1 cup Greek yogurt
1 cup unsalted butter, melted
½ cup sliced almonds
powdered sugar, for dusting
1 cup Greek yogurt, extra

macerated strawberries

2 cups strawberries, sliced
1 tbsp lemon juice
1 tbsp sugar

1 Preheat oven to 350°F (180°C). Grease a 9in (23cm) springform pan. Cut a 9in (23cm) circle of parchment paper to line the bottom of the pan.

2 In a large bowl, combine the sugar, vanilla, eggs, yogurt, and butter. Beat until light and fluffy. Add the flour, baking soda, baking powder, and salt, mixing until well combined. Fold in the strawberries. Spoon the mixture into the pan, smooth the surface, sprinkle with almonds.

3 Bake the cake for 50 minutes or until a skewer inserted into the center comes out clean; cover loosely with foil halfway through baking if the almonds are getting too brown. Leave cake in the pan for 10 minutes. Release the ring; transfer the cake to a wire rack to cool.

4 Meanwhile, make the macerated strawberries. Combine the ingredients in a small bowl; let stand for 20 minutes.

5 Top the cake with the macerated strawberries and dust with powdered sugar; serve with the extra yogurt.

TIP

The cake and macerated strawberries are best made on the day of serving.

Honey vanilla custard pots with phyllo crunch

PREP + COOK TIME **40 MINUTES + REFRIGERATION AND COOLING** | SERVES **4**

Phyllo dough is layered in sheets with butter and bakes up with a delicate, paper-thin result. Its name derives from the Greek word for leaf. Used for making pastries both sweet and savory, here the crunchy phyllo contrasts with the smooth, silky honey custard. You may replace the figs with ripe strawberries, raspberries, or your favorite stone fruit, if you prefer.

¼ cup honey
2 cups milk
1 vanilla bean, split lengthwise
2 tbsp cornstarch (see tip)
1 tbsp brown sugar
1 sheet phyllo dough, 14 x 18in (36 x 46cm)
olive oil cooking spray
2 tbsp finely chopped unsalted pistachios
1 tbsp honey, extra, warmed
4 medium fresh figs, quartered

1. Place honey, milk, and vanilla bean in a medium saucepan over medium heat; bring to a simmer.
2. Whisk the cornstarch and sugar in a medium heat-resistant bowl until combined. Gradually whisk the warm milk mixture into the cornstarch mixture, smoothing out any lumps; return to the pan. Bring to a boil, whisking constantly, until the mixture boils and thickens. Discard the vanilla bean.
3. Pour the mixture into four 1-cup serving glasses or dishes. Refrigerate for 2 hours or until chilled and firm.
4. Meanwhile, preheat oven to 350°F (180°C). Line a baking sheet with parchment paper.
5. Place the phyllo dough on a work surface; spray with cooking spray. Sprinkle two-thirds of the pistachios over the pastry. Fold the pastry in half crosswise; brush with extra honey, sprinkle with the remaining pistachios. Bake for 8 minutes or until golden and crisp; cool. Break into pieces.
6. Serve the custards topped with the figs and filo crunch, drizzled with a little more honey, if you like.

TIP

Cornstarch is a thickening agent to make the dessert set. You may substitute tapioca powder instead.

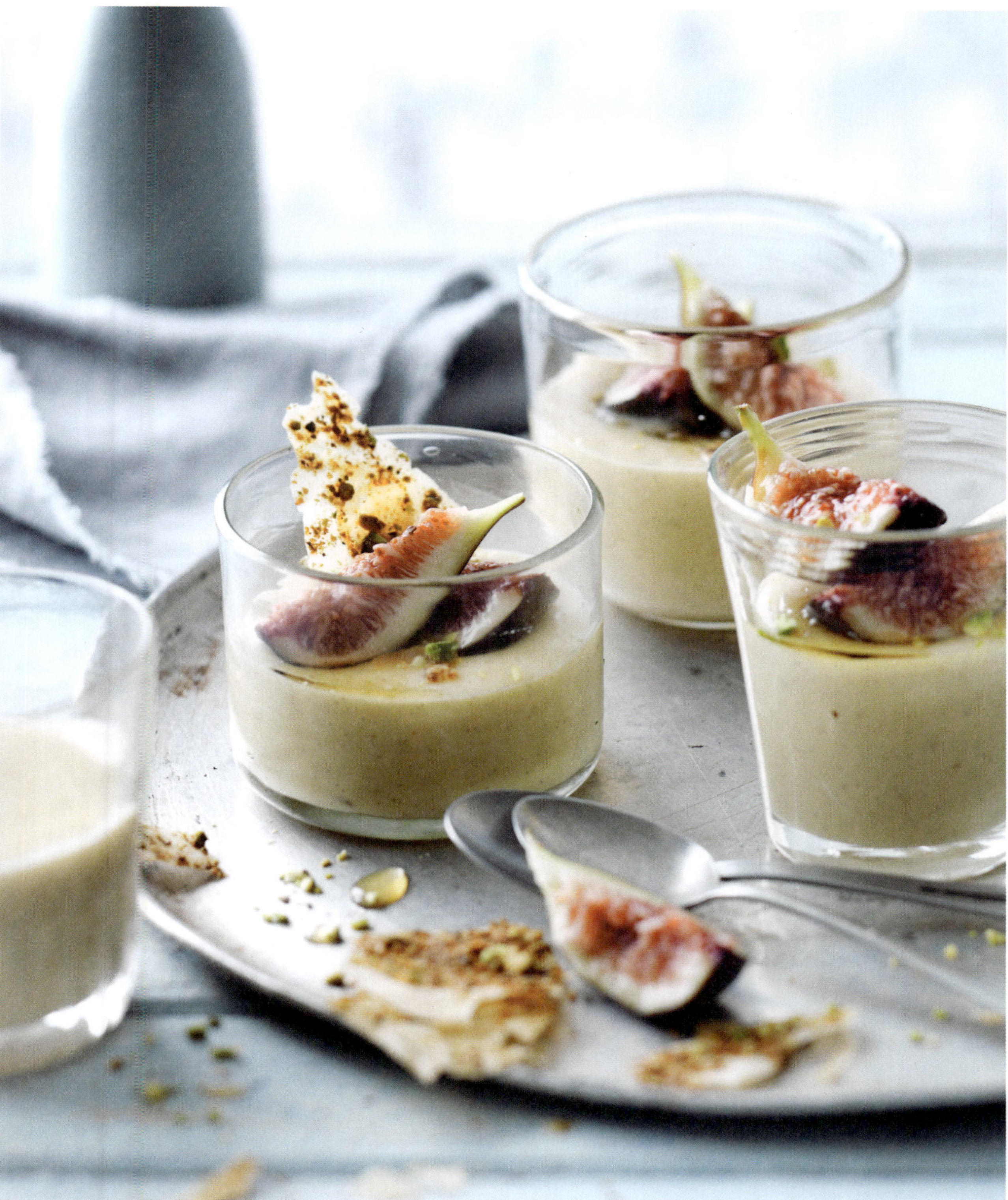

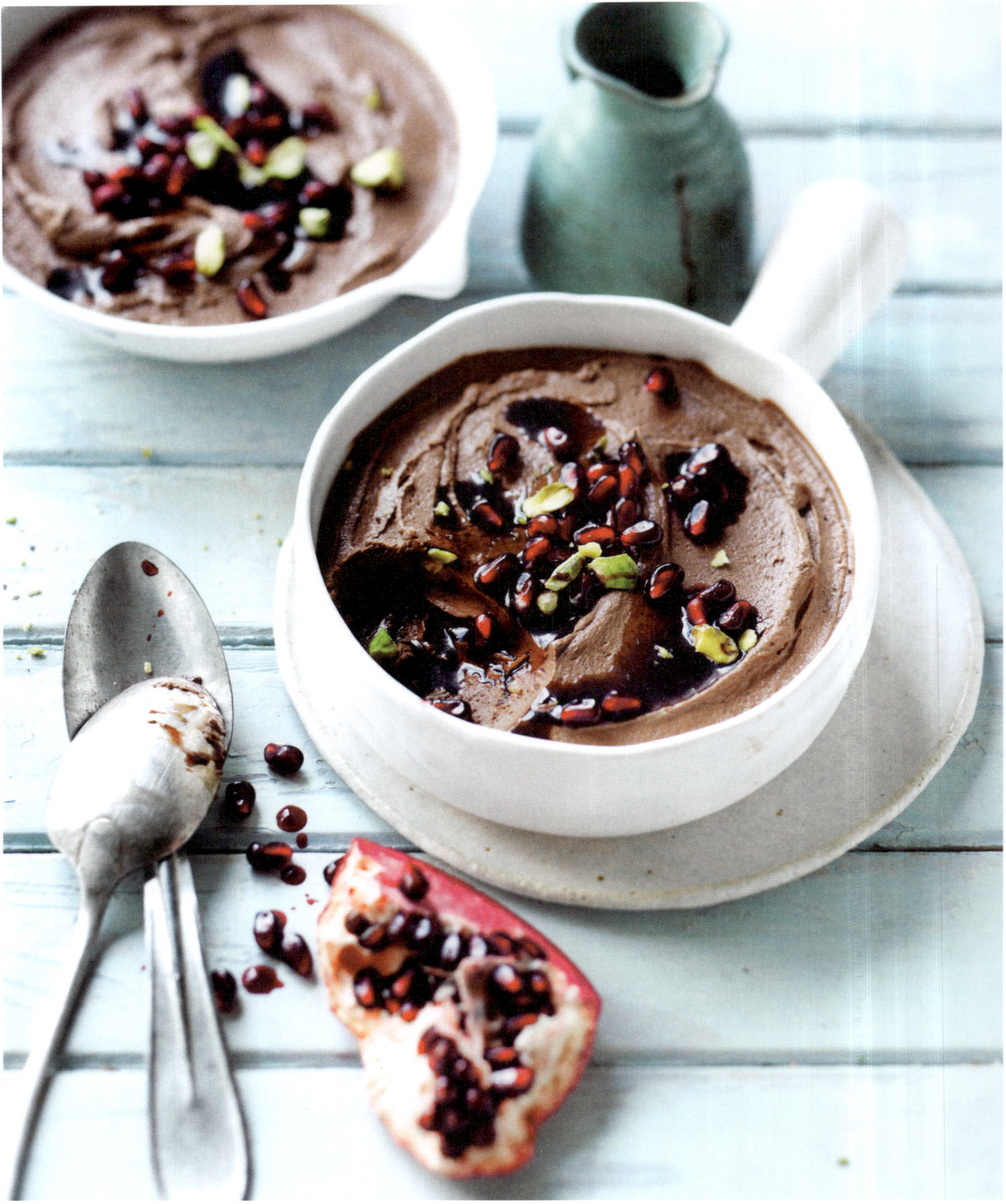

Dark chocolate and ricotta cheese mousse

PREP + COOK TIME **20 MINUTES + COOLING** | SERVES **6**

The rule of thumb for chocolate is that the higher the percentage of cocoa, the better it is for you. Quality dark chocolate is rich in fiber and iron, and is a great source of antioxidants. While you shouldn't be eating large quantities of chocolate in one sitting because it's high in sugar and calories, a bit of dark chocolate in your diet is a great sweet treat.

$1/4$ cup honey
1 tbsp cocoa powder, unsweetened
$1/2$ tsp vanilla extract
$1\frac{1}{2}$ cups dark chocolate (70% cocoa), coarsely chopped
6 fresh dates, pitted
$1/2$ cup milk
2 cups soft ricotta cheese
2 tbsp pomegranate seeds (see tips)
2 tbsp chopped pistachios

1. Make the cocoa syrup. Stir the honey, cocoa, vanilla extract, and 2 tbsp water in a small saucepan over medium heat; bring to a boil. Let cool.
2. Place the chocolate in a small heat-resistant bowl over a small saucepan of simmering water (don't let the water touch the base of the bowl); stir until melted and smooth.
3. In the bowl of a food processor, add the dates and milk. Pulse until the dates are finely chopped. Add the ricotta cheese, process until smooth. Add the melted chocolate; process until well combined to make the mousse.
4. Spoon the mousse evenly into six $3/4$ cup serving bowls or glasses. Spoon the cocoa syrup on the mousse; top with the pomegranate seeds and pistachios.

TIP

Fresh pomegranate seeds are sometimes found in the refrigerated section of the produce department. If they're not available, see page 131 for instructions on how to remove them from the fruit. Alternatively, top each serving with fresh cherries instead.

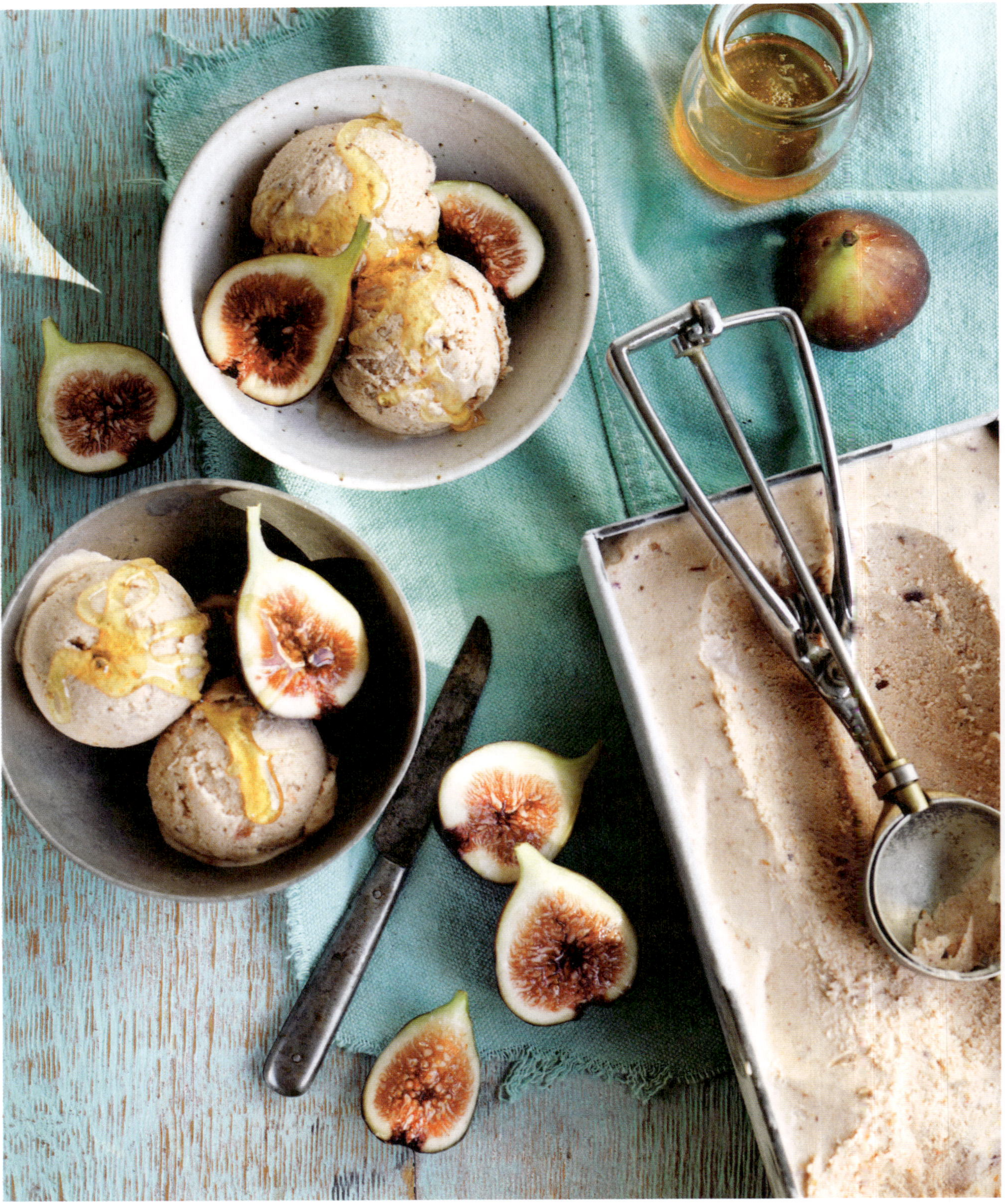

Roasted fig and yogurt ice cream

PREP + COOK TIME **45 MINUTES + COOLING AND FREEZING** | SERVES **8**

This is more of a frozen yogurt, so it's less creamy than traditional ice cream. Since it's lower in fat, it's a healthier choice. Greek yogurt is rich in probiotics, the live bacteria and yeasts that are good for your health, especially your digestive system. The probiotic found in yogurt is known as lactobacillus, and it helps breaks down lactose.

12 large ripe figs, halved
3/4 cup brown sugar
2 tsp finely grated orange zest
1/3 cup freshly squeezed orange juice
3 cups Greek yogurt
2/3 cup crème fraîche (see tip)
1/3 cup honey, plus extra to serve
6 ripe figs, extra, halved

1. Preheat oven to 425°F (220°C). Line a baking sheet with parchment paper.
2. Place the figs, sugar, orange zest, and orange juice in a bowl; toss to combine. Spread the figs on the baking sheet in one layer, cut-side up; roast for 15 minutes or until tender and bubbling. Let cool for 10 minutes.
3. Line a 9in (23cm) loaf pan with parchment paper, extending the paper over the long sides.
4. In a large bowl, combine the yogurt, crème fraîche, and honey in a large bowl; gently fold in the caramelized figs and the fig roasting juices. Spoon the mixture into the lined pan. Freeze for 4 hours or until partially frozen.
5. Remove from freezer. Roughly chop the mixture. Place in a large food processor bowl, pulse to break up the ice crystals. Return to the pan. Freeze for 4 hours or until firm.
6. Let the ice cream stand at room temperature for 10 minutes to soften slightly before serving. Serve it topped with the extra figs; drizzle with extra honey.

TIPS

- You may substitute sour cream or mascarpone for the crème fraîche.
- If you have an ice cream maker, this mixture can be churned following the manufacturer's instructions.
- Store leftover ice cream in the freezer for up to 1 month.

Citrus yogurt cups

PREP + COOK TIME **45 MINUTES** | SERVES **4**

In the dark, cold months of winter, the only bright spot is the copious ripe, juicy citrus fruits that come into season. While it's well known that citrus fruits are an excellent source of vitamin C, which helps boost your immune system in cold and flu season, they also have other health benefits. The antioxidant-rich red grapefruit, for example, helps lower cholesterol.

1 vanilla bean
⅓ cup sugar
6 wide strips orange zest (see tip)
1 tbsp orange juice
3 small clementines, peeled, sliced horizontally (see tip)
1 medium ruby grapefruit, peeled, segmented
3 cups Greek yogurt
small fresh mint leaves, to garnish

1 Split the vanilla bean in half lengthwise; scrape seeds into a small saucepan. Add the vanilla pod, sugar, orange zest, and ½ cup water to the pan; bring to a boil. Reduce heat to low; cook for 6 minutes or until the syrup has thickened slightly. Cool. Discard the vanilla bean pod; stir in the orange juice.

2 Combine the clementine slices, grapefruit segments, and sugar syrup in a medium bowl.

3 Spoon the yogurt into four 1¼-cup serving glasses. Top with the citrus mixture and mint.

TIPS

- For orange strips, use a vegetable peeler to peel wide strips; avoid taking off too much of the white pith with the rind, as it's bitter.
- You may use tangerines instead of clementines.
- The syrup can be made 4 hours ahead and combined with the citrus; refrigerate until needed.

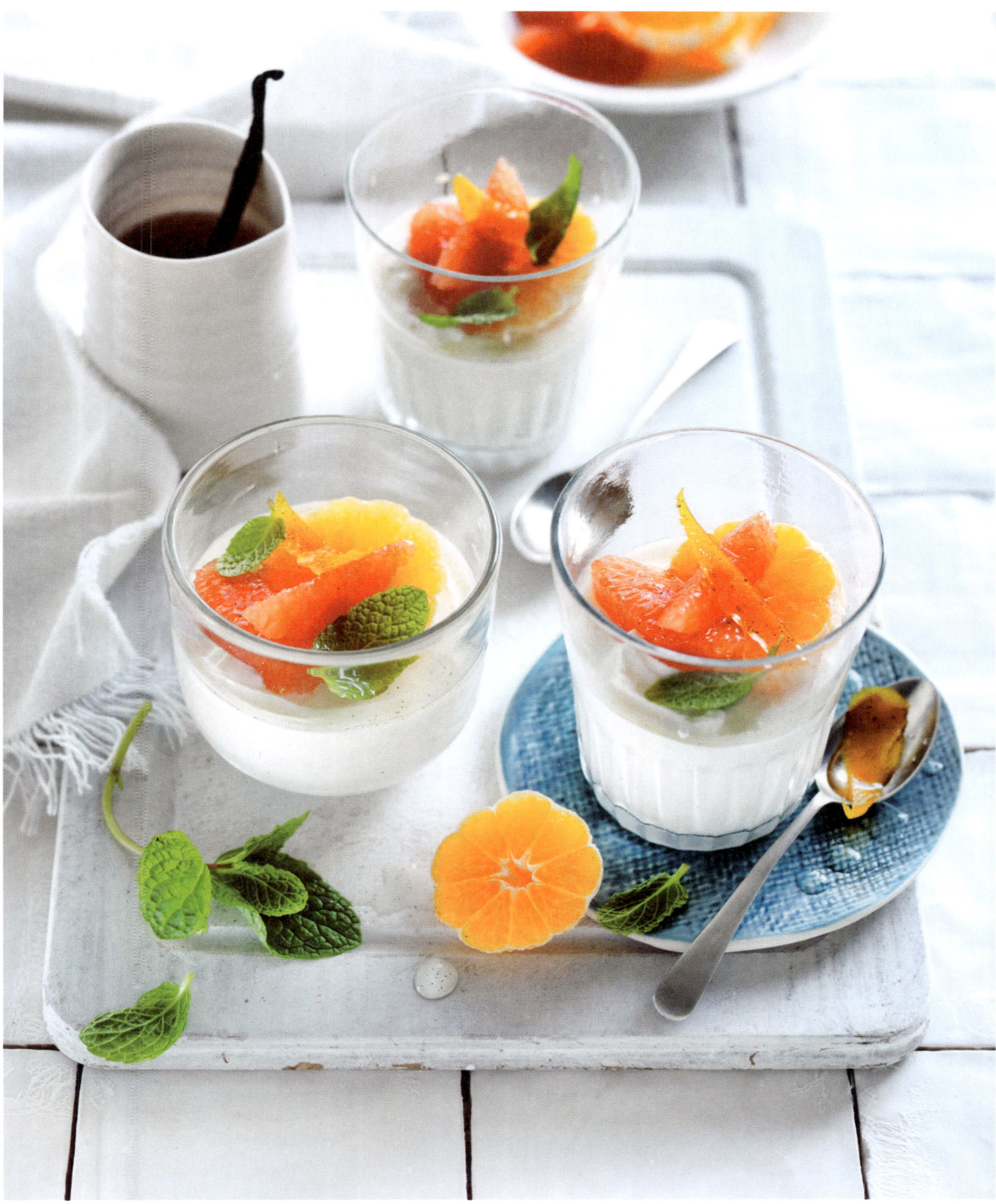

Honey-baked peaches and grapes with sweet ricotta cheese

PREP + COOK TIME **40 MINUTES** | SERVES **4**

There is no more straightforward dessert than baked fruit. Their bright, sweet flavors are amplified to become a delicious warming dish, which is healthy to boot. Accompanied here with a sweetened ricotta cheese, the fruit could also be served with ice cream, crème fraîche, or creamy Greek yogurt. Or use the fruit and syrup as a topper for a plain cake.

6 medium peaches, pitted, quartered (see tips)
1lb (450g) seedless red grapes, halved
1 tbsp honey
4 sprigs fresh thyme, plus extra to serve
1½ cups firm ricotta cheese
2 tbsp sugar
½ tsp finely grated orange zest, plus extra to serve

1. Preheat oven to 400°F (200°C). Line a baking sheet with parchment paper.
2. Place the peaches and grapes on the baking sheet; drizzle with honey and top with thyme. Bake for 25 minutes or until tender and syrupy.
3. Meanwhile, mix the ricotta cheese, sugar, and orange zest until smooth.
4. Serve the baked fruit and any cooking juices with the ricotta mixture, topped with the extra orange zest and fresh thyme.

TIPS

- Use plums instead of peaches, if you like.
- This dish can be served for brunch or dessert. It also travels well, so it's a great addition to a picnic basket. Pack the ricotta cheese and fruit separately; keep the ricotta cheese cold.

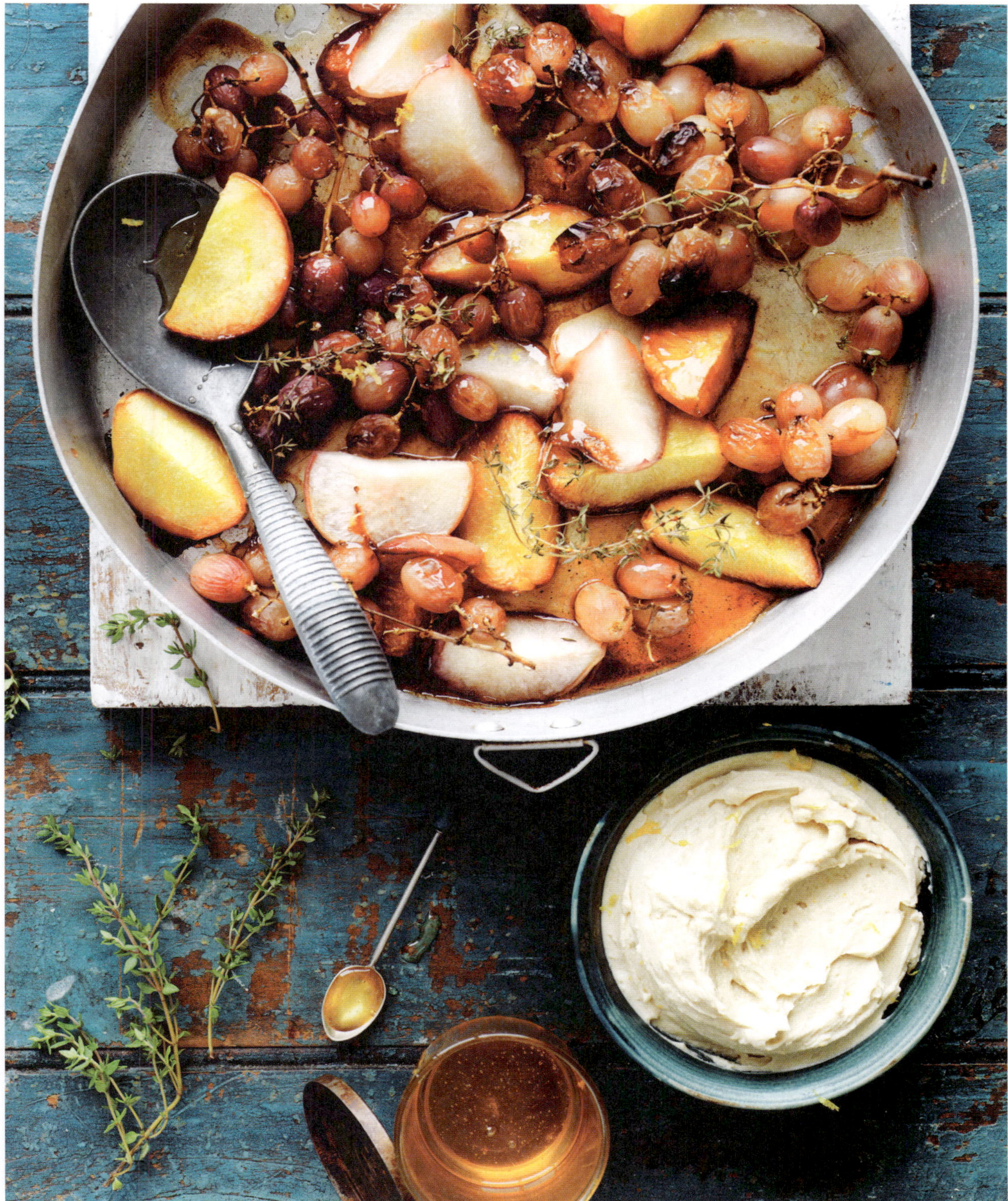

Baked ricotta cheese pudding with orange syrup and cherries

PREP + COOK TIME **1 HOUR + COOLING AND REFRIGERATION** | SERVES **4**

Humans have collected honey since ancient times. In the absence of sugar, it's used as a sweetener in many traditional desserts in the Mediterranean region. The earliest record of honey harvesting is in an 8,000-year-old cave painting in Valencia, Spain, which depicts two figures using a ladder to gather the sweet liquid from high beehives.

3½ cups fresh ricotta cheese
4 eggs
½ cup honey
¾ tsp ground cinnamon
2 tsp finely grated orange zest
½ cup fresh cherries, pitted
2 tbsp coarsely chopped pistachios, to serve

orange syrup
zest of 1 orange, finely grated
½ cup orange juice
½ cup honey
1 cinnamon stick
½ tsp fresh thyme leaves

1. Preheat oven to 350°F (180°C). Butter a 4-cup heatproof casserole
2. In the bowl of a food processor, combine the ricotta cheese, eggs, honey, cinnamon, and orange zest. Pulse until smooth. Pour the mixture evenly into the dish.
3. Bake the pudding for 30 minutes or until the center is just firm to touch. Cool to room temperature. Refrigerate for 1 hour or until cold.
4. Meanwhile, make the orange syrup. Combine the orange zest, orange juice, honey, water, cinnamon stick, thyme leaves, and ½ cup water in a small saucepan; bring to a boil. Reduce heat to low; cook for 10 minutes or until syrupy. Refrigerate for 1 hour or until cold.
5. Serve the pudding topped with the cherries, orange syrup, and pistachios.

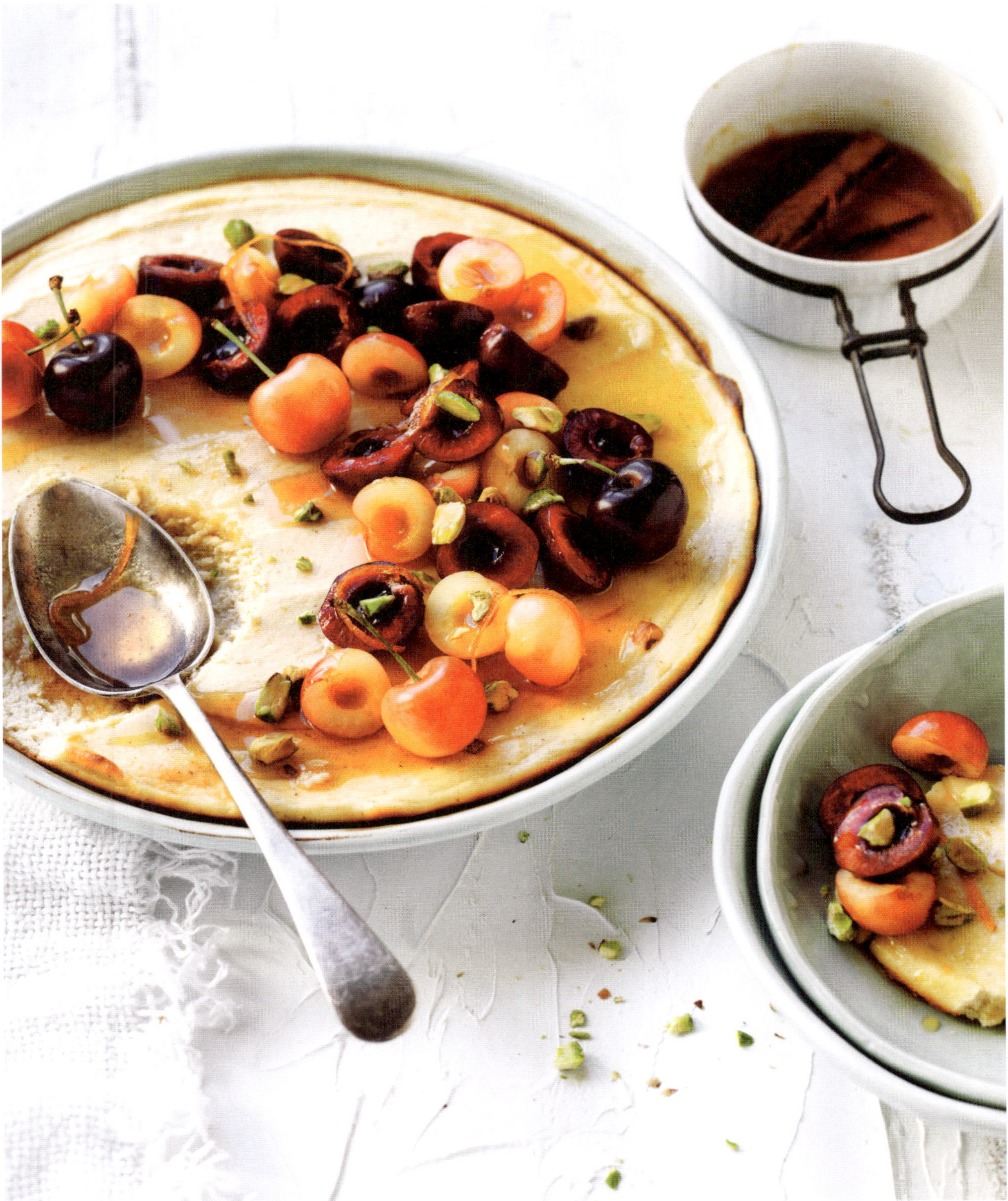

Conversion chart

A note on Australian measures used to develop these recipes

- One Australian metric measuring cup holds approximately 250ml, whereas a US cup holds 237ml.
- One Australian metric tablespoon holds 20ml, whereas a US tablespoon holds 14.7 ml.
- One Australian metric teaspoon holds 5ml, whereas a US teaspoon holds 4.9 ml.
- The difference between one country's measuring cups and another's is within a two-or three-teaspoon variance, and should not affect your cooking results.

Using measures in this book

- All cup and spoon measurements are level.
- The most accurate way of measuring dry ingredients is to weigh them.
- When measuring liquids, use a clear glass or measuring cup with metric markings.
- We use large eggs with an average weight of 60g.

Dry measures

metric	imperial
15g	1/2oz
30g	1oz
60g	2oz
90g	3oz
125g	4oz (1/4lb)
155g	5oz
185g	6oz
220g	7oz
250g	8oz (1/2lb)
280g	9oz
315g	10oz
345g	11oz
375g	12oz (3/4lb)
410g	13oz
440g	14oz
470g	15oz
500g	16oz (1lb)
750g	24oz (1 1/2lb)
1kg	32oz (2lb)

Liquid measures

metric	imperial
30ml	1 fluid oz
60ml	2 fluid oz
100ml	3 fluid oz
125ml	4 fluid oz
150ml	5 fluid oz
190ml	6 fluid oz
250ml	8 fluid oz
300ml	10 fluid oz
500ml	16 fluid oz
600ml	20 fluid oz
1000ml (1 liter)	1 3/4 pints

Length measures

metric	imperial
3mm	1/8in
6mm	1/4in
1cm	1/2in
2cm	3/4in
2.5cm	1in
5cm	2in
6cm	2 1/2in
8cm	3in
10cm	4in
13cm	5in
15cm	6in
18cm	7in
20cm	8in
22cm	9in
25cm	10in
28cm	11in
30cm	12in (1ft)

Oven temperatures

The oven temperatures in this book are for conventional ovens; if you have a convection oven, decrease the temperature by 10–20 degrees.

°F (Fahrenheit)	°C (Celsius)
250	120
300	150
325	160
350	180
400	200
425	220
475	240

Index

Acknowledgments

DK would like to thank Sophia Young, Simone Aquilina, Amanda Chebatte, and Georgia Moore for their assistance in making this book, and Lyndi Cohen for the introductory text.

The Australian Women's Weekly Test Kitchen in Sydney, Australia, developed, tested, and photographed the recipes in this book.